Helping Your Child with Worry and Anxiety

Ann Cox is a CAMHS consultant nurse and clinical lead. She is a CBT therapist, an independent prescriber, a doctoral scholar, and an Associate Editor for Journal of Child Health Care. Ann is also a Florence Nightingale & RCN Foundatio Scholar, the winner of the PPiMH Award 2019 and a Nursing T s Award 2019 finalist. She is passionate about direct clinical work with cl en, young people and families.

Th uthor would like to thank the following for their contributions:

Dr Kristina Keeley-Jones

San hor son

Ben ea

Dr aure e Baldwin

Del sia McKnight

Sco t Lunn

Lis Dale

Dr uth Fishwick

Le n Benson

Le ne Walker

A s Bullock

D1331409

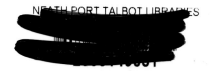

NEATH PORT TALBOT LIBRARIES

Overcoming Common Problems Series

Selected titles

A full list of titles is available from Sheldon Press on our website at
www.sheldonpress.co.uk

Lists of titles in the Mindful Way and Sheldon Short Guides series are also available from Sheldon Press.

Overcoming Common Problems

Helping your Child with Worry and Anxiety

ANN COX

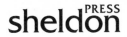

First published by Sheldon Press in 2021
An imprint of John Murray Press
A division of Hodder & Stoughton Ltd,
An Hachette UK company

1

Copyright © Ann Cox 2021

The right of Ann Cox to be identified as the Author of the Work has been
asserted by her in accordance with the Copyright, Designs and Patents Act
1988.

The acknowledgments on pp. i constitute an extension of this copyright page.

All rights reserved. No part of this publication may be reproduced, stored in
a retrieval system, or transmitted, in any form or by any means without the
prior written permission of the publisher, nor be otherwise circulated in any
form of binding or cover other than that in which it is published and without
a similar condition being imposed on the subsequent purchaser.

This book is for information or educational purposes only and is not intended
to act as a substitute for medical advice or treatment. Any person with a
condition requiring medical attention should consult a qualified medical
practitioner or suitable therapist.

A CIP catalogue record for this title is available from the British Library

Trade Paperback ISBN 9781529344455
eBook ISBN 9781529344455

Typeset by KnowledgeWorks Global Ltd.

Printed and bound in Great Britain by Clays Ltd, Elcograf S.p.A.

John Murray Press policy is to use papers that are natural, renewable and
recyclable products and made from wood grown in sustainable forests. The
logging and manufacturing processes are expected to conform to the envi-
ronmental regulations of the country of origin.

John Murray Press
Carmelite House
50 Victoria Embankment
London EC4Y 0DZ

NEATH PORT TALBOT LIBRARIES	
2300149031	
Askews & Holts	23-Aug-2021
618.928	£10.99
NPTPON	

To my Husband Ellis and Daughter Jessica, this book would not have been possible without your constant patience and inspiration.

For every child who is struggling with worries or anxieties, and for every parent who is supporting them, this book is for you, in offering hope, strategies and a better future.

Contents

1
Anxiety

Ann Cox, RMN & CBT Therapist

This chapter provides an overview of what anxiety is. It will help you understand the nature of anxiety in the body, why a range of anxiety difficulties present with similar symptoms and, most importantly, how these symptoms can be managed by your child and within the family setting. Understanding what anxiety is is core to managing the range of anxiety difficulties discussed in this book.

Anxiety as an umbrella term

Anxiety is an umbrella term for a range of different difficulties. Here are some of the difficulties that come under the 'anxiety umbrella'.

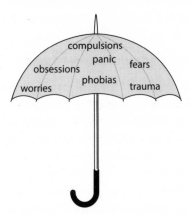

Figure 1.1 Difficulties under the 'anxiety umbrella'

How common is anxiety?

Anxiety disorders are one of the most common disorders in children and young people. According to data collected by NHS

Digital (2017), children are three times more likely to struggle with anxiety than depression. In 5–10-year-olds, around four in every 100 children will have anxiety. For 11–16-year-olds, it is approximately eight in every 100 girls and six in every 100 boys. For girls aged 17–19 years of age it is approximately 13 in every 100, in contrast to around five in every 100 boys of the same age (NHS Digital, 2017). A follow-up study by NHS Digital in 2020 suggested that the increase in mental health disorders of children increased by 16 per cent across all disorders. However, this further study was undertaken during the 2020 pandemic of COVID-19 (NHS Digital, 2020), so there may be unusually high figures reported here.

Anxiety affects children. Not all of these children will seek help, as some children may be able to manage their anxiety despite it being difficult. There are many resources on the internet and apps that are easily accessible for children to use as guided self-help. As with most mental health difficulties, the earlier you start to treat the anxiety, the better the outcome. If your child is struggling with anxiety, wherever possible, get help as soon as you can to ensure the earliest and best possible outcome.

Psycho-education of anxiety

The art of explaining how anxiety works in the body is called psycho-education. Psycho-education should be the first intervention offered to any child. Psycho-education can have a very positive impact. If your child can understand how anxiety works in their body and what they need to do to manage it, it may be the only intervention they need. The rest of this chapter focuses on psycho-education, to help you explain to your child what anxiety is in a way that they can understand.

Common symptoms are present across all the different anxiety difficulties as illustrated in Figure 1.3. These symptoms will differ in number and intensity for each child. One reason why there are common symptoms in all of these difficulties, is because the symptoms are activated through a single physiological pathway in the body. This means that the same chain of events happens in the body every time a child becomes anxious.

What is anxiety?

Q: Does anxiety make a child feel worried, panicky, scared or nervous?
A: Yes, it can. These are the feelings people describe when asked to describe anxiety.
Q: Can anxiety can be helpful?
A: Yes, it is helpful: anxiety is needed to protect us.

Anxiety symptoms are experienced as result of the in-built threat system in the brain being activated. For the majority of the time, this threat system works to help us complete everyday tasks like crossing a road, cutting vegetables with a knife, or navigating some steep steps. It does this by alerting us to potential danger. We look to cross the road when it is clear to ensure no harm comes to us; we ensure our fingers are out of the way when we are cutting vegetables; and we ensure the safe placement of our feet when we are navigating steep or difficult ground. Our threat system and anxiety symptoms can help us manage things that can be challenging and which may lead to harm if we are not careful. Anxiety, and the threat system, are primarily developed to keep us safe. However, sometimes the threat system can become too sensitive and this is where anxiety can become unhelpful and impact on many areas of life.

How does anxiety work in the body?

The threat system is also known as the fight-or-flight system. The fight-or-flight system is like an alarm that has been set off in our brains, telling us we are in potential danger. The alarm sets off a chain of events that will result in anxiety symptoms. The symptoms of anxiety help to get the body ready for action, to either run away from the threatening situation (*flight*) or to stay and *fight* the threat. On some occasions, people may be so overcome with these symptoms that they freeze with fear. These are known as the 3Fs: *fight*, *flight* and *freeze*. When the threat system in the brain is activated, the fight-or-flight system is triggered.

The brain senses a threat or danger. It sends a message through the autonomic nervous system to activate the fight or flight response.

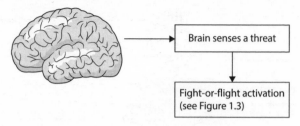

Figure 1.2 Anxiety chain of events

The fight-or-flight system has been part of our brains for hundreds of thousands of years and can be traced back to the cave people. Our brains developed the threat system to protect us, as the environment at that time had many predators and potential threats. Predators included animals such as bears and sabretooth tigers, snakes and poisonous spiders, and threats such as difficult terrain, high cliffs, mud and landslides. The fight-or-flight threat system was much needed at this time to help keep us safe.

The world has changed enormously since prehistoric times, and now we have so many other things that help keep us safe. We have simple things such as clothes and shoes, signs to alert us to potential danger, railings and fences to keep us safe from falling, we have alarms on lorries when they are reversing so we can hear the danger coming, we have media, news and telecommunications; we have so many systems that alert us to danger. But despite the world around us evolving and changing, our brains still have the same threat system we developed hundreds of thousands of years ago. Sometimes this threat system can get over sensitive and this is why we start to experience too much anxiety, and it can become a problem.

What happens in our body when fight-or-flight is activated?

When our fight or flight system is activated, it increases the levels of two hormones in our body: **noradrenaline** and **adrenaline**. These hormones set off a common chain of events in the body, including:

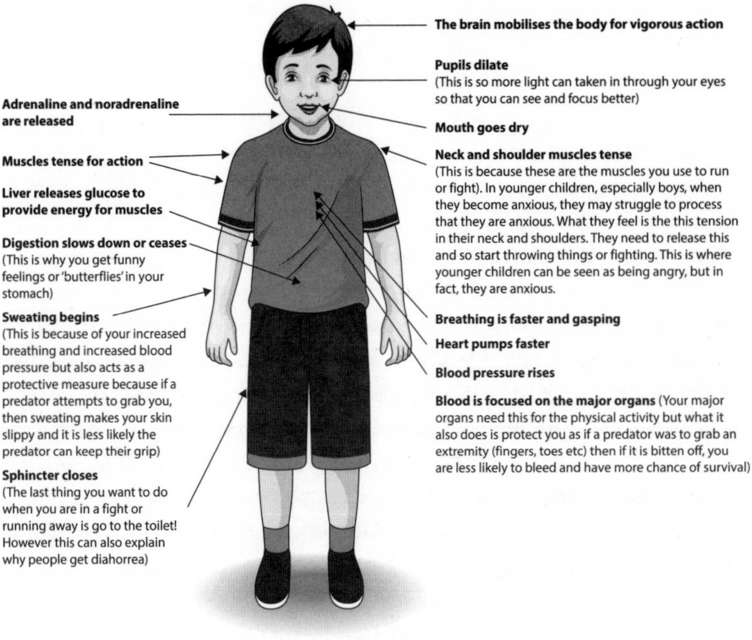

The brain mobilises the body for vigorous action

Pupils dilate
(This is so more light can taken in through your eyes so that you can see and focus better)

Adrenaline and noradrenaline are released

Mouth goes dry

Muscles tense for action

Neck and shoulder muscles tense
(This is because these are the muscles you use to run or fight). In younger children, especially boys, when they become anxious, they may struggle to process that they are anxious. What they feel is the this tension in their neck and shoulders. They need to release this and so start throwing things or fighting. This is where younger children can be seen as being angry, but in fact, they are anxious.

Liver releases glucose to provide energy for muscles

Digestion slows down or ceases
(This is why you get funny feelings or 'butterflies' in your stomach)

Breathing is faster and gasping

Heart pumps faster

Sweating begins
(This is because of your increased breathing and increased blood pressure but also acts as a protective measure because if a predator attempts to grab you, then sweating makes your skin slippy and it is less likely the predator can keep their grip)

Blood pressure rises

Blood is focused on the major organs (Your major organs need this for the physical activity but what it also does is protect you as if a predator was to grab an extremity (fingers, toes etc) then if it is bitten off, you are less likely to bleed and have more chance of survival)

Sphincter closes
(The last thing you want to do when you are in a fight or running away is go to the toilet! However this can also explain why people get diahorrea)

Figure 1.3 Fight-or-flight symptoms (anxiety)

One fantastic thing that you need to know about the human body is that, when it is healthy, one of its main functions is to keep harmony, to stay in balance. If the body is off balance in any way, then it will try to rebalance itself, a little bit like trying to get a see-saw level. This is called *homeostasis* (from the Latin *homeo* meaning 'man' and *stasis* meaning 'static'). To maintain homeostasis, for example, the body will level up sugars and fats in the body when you have eaten or drunk, keep your temperature regular, keep your vitamins and hormones at the right levels. Your body is doing this all the time without you knowing, in a bid to stay healthy. For some people, there will be complications if some part of the body is not working properly. Diabetics, for example, cannot control their blood sugars because their pancreas is not working properly, so medication is usually needed to help maintain homeostasis. The process of homeostasis takes approximately 40 minutes and the action of homeostasis is important in the role of anxiety.

We can think of the activation of the fight-or-flight system as the 'up' system (the biological name is the *sympathetic nervous system*). As we have seen previously, whenever the body is unbalanced, as it would be in fight or flight when we have higher levels of adrenaline and noradrenaline, the body tries to create balance through the function of homeostasis. We can think of this process as the 'down' system (the biological name is the *parasympathetic nervous system* – I remember this by associating *para* with a 'parachute' bringing the fight-or-flight system down). The 'down' system is also known as the 'rest and digest' process, as the body returns to rest (from the fight or flight) and the digestion process starts working again. What is also known about the 'down' system is that we can help its action by contributing to some of the things it is trying to achieve. For example, the 'down' system will try and regulate breathing as the 'up' system will have increased it. If breathing is regulated by your child, this will help the progress of the down system. Breathing exercises, like breathing as if you are pretending to blow up a balloon, will help.

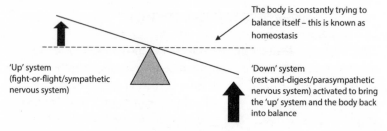

The body is constantly trying to balance itself – this is known as homeostasis

'Up' system (fight-or-flight/sympathetic nervous system)

'Down' system (rest-and-digest/parasympathetic nervous system) activated to bring the 'up' system and the body back into balance

Figure 1.4 See-saw of up-and-down system

Once the 'up' system has been activated, the 'down' system will automatically be activated, too. This creates homeostasis and brings the noradrenaline and adrenaline down to their normal levels in the body, and takes about 40 minutes. This is important to know: over the period of 40 minutes, your anxiety symptoms *will come down on their own*. You do not have to do anything to make this happen, it is how the body is designed to keep itself healthy. If your child is anxious, they may think that they are anxious all day and that there is no relief from the anxiety; biologically, however, this is impossible.

Having your child test this out to see if it works is really helpful, as they can make the connection with what is happening in their body, and how it reduces anxiety on its own. A good way to do this is for your child to think of something that makes them a little bit scared, but is not overwhelming for them. So if we were to think of a 0–10 scale of anxiety, with 0 being no anxiety at all, and 10 being the most anxiety anyone could feel, they should think of something that raises their anxiety to between a 6 and an 8. You may have to work with the child to find a source of anxiety that works for them – perhaps, for example, they are apprehensive about spiders, or crane flies. You could test out homeostasis with them by asking your child to go near to the spider, or whatever else they have chosen, to stay close to it, and to see what happens to their anxiety by measuring it every five minutes. It's helpful to use a quick and easy table (below) to record the level of anxiety after each five-minute period.

Minutes	Level of anxiety
0	
5	
10	
15	
20	
25	
30	
35	
40	

By testing anxiety out in this way, as long as your child is concentrating on the object that is making them anxious (rather than something else), their anxiety level will gradually come down over the 40 minutes. This is called 'habituation'. In order to successfully reduce anxiety, there is a need to habituate to whatever is making you anxious. Of course, habituation cannot work when a child is avoiding the object that is making them anxious, either physically or mentally.

Physical avoidance is something we all do. It is an easy and safe way to avoid something challenging. However, when avoidance of an object starts to impact on life, it becomes a problem. Figure 1.5 shows what happens when a child avoids an object. We can use the spider analogy to describe this, because it's easy for most people to associate with and we'll use the story of Jessica, who was afraid of spiders. The first time Jessica went to the bathroom and saw a big spider in the bath, her level of anxiety went up to a 10: this is the first arrow, going from 0 up to 10. In the bathroom, Jessica screamed, ran out of the bathroom, shut the door and shouted for her parents to come and help. Because Jessica ran away (*flight*) and avoided the spider (rather than stay with it, as we would with habituation), her anxiety reduced back down to 0 because the spider was no longer deemed a threat. When she did the same thing again on other occasions (time 2, 3 and 4), Jessica's anxiety repeated the same action as it did previously, and went to 10 out of 10. As Jessica repeated the same actions and avoided the spider, her anxiety responded in exactly the same way. Whenever children avoid anxiety, the same response is likely to be experienced.

What Jessica has learned is that when she avoids things that make her anxious, her anxiety will reduce. However her level of anxiety will feel in the same situation on different occasions, Jessica will always have a 10/10 response, and this is unlikely to change if the same actions are taken each time.

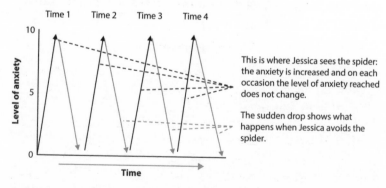

This is where Jessica sees the spider: the anxiety is increased and on each occasion the level of anxiety reached does not change.

The sudden drop shows what happens when Jessica avoids the spider.

Figure 1.5 Graph to show what happens in the avoidance of anxiety

Habituation, on the other hand, does change the level of anxiety experienced. When children test out or expose themselves to the object that makes them anxious and stay with it, the anxiety will eventually lessen in severity and will occur for a shorter length of time. The graph below shows how this happens.

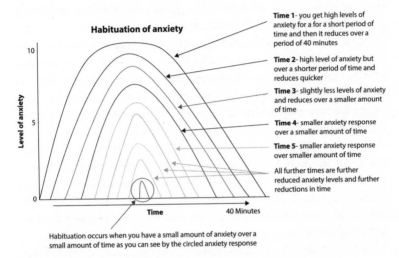

Figure 1.6 Graph to show what happens in habituation

Habituation is something that needs to be done frequently to ensure that the level of anxiety remains low. If we stop habituating and start avoiding, the anxiety levels will increase again.

Safety behaviours

'Safety behaviours' are things that we do to make ourselves feel better when we are in anxiety-provoking situations. Perhaps we are waiting in a queue where there are number of other people; this may cause us anxiety, especially if we are anxious about other people's judgement. We may use behaviours to make us feel better in that situation: looking at our mobile phones, searching in bags for things and so avoiding eye contact with people, staring at the floor or listening to music through headphones. Whilst safety behaviours can make us feel safe, sometimes they can be unhelpful. One type of unhelpful safety behaviour used a lot by children is reassurance (or seeking reassurance).

Reassurance

Reassurance is something we should all provide for our children. Children are vulnerable and by offering reassurance, as parents, we are providing guidance and support to help our children develop and take risks to increase their independence. If you think about the first time your child took an independent step, or when your child tries a new activity, of course you offer them reassurance. Reassurance is important to everyone. However at times, especially in anxiety, reassurance can be unhelpful. Too much reassurance can be counterproductive and become part of the anxiety cycle rather than reducing the anxiety.

Let us think about Jessica again, but this time in a slightly different situation. This time, Jessica has worries about things that are going to happen. She worries about school, she worries about her friendships and she worries about her grandma. Every time Jessica has a worry, she tells her mum about it and asks her mum whether everything is going to be alright. Her mum reassures Jessica and says, yes, everything is going to be alright. What happens here is that Jessica has a thought, her level of anxiety is increasing, she asks her mum for reassurance, her mum gives her reassurance and Jessica's anxiety goes down. The next time Jessica has a worry, the same process happens again, and the same outcome happens again. Jessica's anxiety about her worries never changes. We can match this response to the avoidance of anxiety cycle in Figure 1.5, because the level of anxiety never changes and Jessica avoids the worry by asking her mum to manage it through reassurance. Reassuring a child that everything will be okay, when potentially it may not be, can cause problems in the future. It is really important that we are as honest as we can be – we can't prevent some things from happening, like the death of a loved one. When there are questions asked, responses such as 'as far as I know' can be more helpful and realistic.

Reassurance includes anything that is preventing your child from being independent, such as having your child sleep in your bed or bedroom (co-sleeping). But often reassurance is unhelpful, and a more useful way to help your child manage the worries that they have is to help them to reassure themselves. This can be done by offering verbal reassurance *once* to your child (as this is a normal, supportive action) but, after this, your child has to learn to reassure themselves. You can support this by changing the responses you give to your child, saying, 'What did I say the last time?' or 'What do you think?', or you could get your child to write the response on a whiteboard or a note and ask them to go and read it when they ask in the future. This helps the child process and manage the worry for themselves and will reduce their anxiety. In some cases it can be incredibly difficult to break the cycle, but it will help reduce the level of anxiety.

Figure 1.7 shows the cycle of reassurance. The blue line is the parent reassuring the child, and the green line represents the child reassuring themselves.

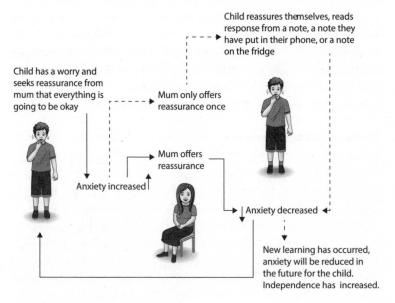

Figure 1.7 Cycle of reassurance

Misinterpretation of symptoms

Misinterpretation of symptoms is really common in children. In Figure 1.3 we gave some of the symptoms of anxiety. Children who have anxiety may often complain of having a headache or a tummy ache, misinterpreting and focussing on one symptom instead of understanding it is from a group of symptoms related to anxiety. It is important to look out for these as a parent.

Other misinterpretations come from other emotions using the same 'up' system as anxiety; these other emotions may have many of the same symptoms as anxiety but are there for a totally different reason. These emotions include feeling excited, feeling angry, the anticipation of having an adrenaline rush from certain activities (like a rollercoaster ride) and, at times, overtiredness can present with similar symptoms. If a child has been experiencing lots of anxiety symptoms the brain starts recognizing these symptoms as anxiety, and it becomes a default setting. Even when the symptoms are not anxiety driven, the brain can default them to anxiety. It can be really common, for example, for a child experiencing something exciting, like a birthday or festive holiday, to have symptoms because they are excited – but they will interpret them as anxiety because that is what the brain has defaulted to. It is really helpful to work through what emotion your child is feeling if this should occur, and to start naming emotions.

Big shout out to nature

Being outside in nature can really help with a sense of wellbeing. Evidence has proven that spending time in nature helps your brain and your body relax. Going for woodland walks, bird and wildlife watching, making dens, visiting streams and rivers will help improve your child's mood, reduce anxiety and improve wellbeing. Getting out in nature will be a great addition to some of the strategies included in this book. The Woodland Trust's website provides lots of fun activities you can do with your child in the woodlands.

Physical health causes of anxiety

Whilst anxiety is common among children, there should always be caution around any physical health issues that may cause anxiety.

Adolescence is a time where there are many hormonal changes in the body and sometimes this can an impact on the child's physical health. The thyroid, a small gland found in the neck which regulates some hormones, can sometimes change its function during adolescence, so it might be important to get this ruled out as a possible cause. Other causes could be vitamin deficiencies, respiratory and cardiac disorders, irritable bowel difficulties and medical conditions related to the fight or flight system. It is important that you contact your GP and ensure any physical reasons for anxiety are ruled out.

Summary

This chapter has provided you with an overview of anxiety, how it works in the body and how you as a parent can help your child manage some of the behaviours that we know children struggle with. It is really helpful to think about how you and your child team up to beat anxiety and stop feeding it on behaviours such as reassurance and avoidance. The rest of this book provides strategies and support in managing specific anxiety difficulties, whilst also ensuring you look after yourself as a parent. Keeping yourself well and in a good frame of mind will undoubtedly help your child.

References and further reading

Lader, M. and Marks, I. (2013) *Clinical Anxiety.* London: William Heinemann.

Moss, S. (2012) *Natural Childhood Report.* [Online]. Available at: <nt. global.ssl.fastly.net/documents/read-our-natural-childhood-report. pdf> (accessed: 1 February 2021).

NHS Digital (2017) *Mental Health of Children and Young People in England, 2017.* [Online]. Available at: <digital.nhs.uk/data-and-information/ publications/statistical/mental-health-of-children-and-young-people-in-england/2017/2017> (accessed: 9 June 2020).

NHS Digital (2020) *Mental Health of Children and Young People in England, 2020.* [Online]. Available at: <files.digital.nhs.uk/CB/C41981/ mhcyp_2020_rep.pdf> (accessed: 25 October 2020).

Online resources

Anxiety UK. *Free anxiety resources.* <www.anxietyuk.org.uk/get-help/free-anxiety-resources/>

Barnardos. *What is anxiety?* <www.barnardos.org.uk/blog/what-anxiety>

MindEd. *MindEd Hub.* <www.minded.org.uk>

NHS. *Anxiety in children.* <www.nhs.uk/conditions/stress-anxiety-depression/anxiety-in-children/>

NHS. *NHS Apps Library.* <www.nhs.uk/apps-library/>

NHS. *Every mind matters.* <www.nhs.uk/oneyou/every-mind-matters/childrens-mental-health/>

Stem4. *Anxiety for teenagers.* <stem4.org.uk/anxiety/anxiety-for-teenagers/>

The Working Together Team. *Might Moe: An Anxiety Workbook for Children.* <website.twtt.org.uk/media/Mighty%20Moe1%20Anxiety.pdf>

Woodland Trust. *Woodland adventures for children and families.* <www.woodlandtrust.org.uk/visiting-woods/things-to-do/children-and-families/>

Young Minds. *Anxiety.* <youngminds.org.uk/find-help/conditions/anxiety/>

2
Looking after yourself as a parent

Ann Cox, RMN & CBT Therapist
Dr Kristina Keeley-Jones, Clinical Psychologist

This chapter is specifically for you as a parent or a caregiver to help you look after yourself. Looking after yourself through self-care is just as important as caring for your child – there is truth in the saying 'you can't pour from an empty cup'. Supporting a child with worries and anxieties is a hard task and it is vital that you keep your cup, and your resilience, as full as you can. We hope this chapter will increase your own self-awareness and give you some great strategies to keep you going through those difficult times. Remember – you can only ever give your best, but to give your best, you need to look after yourself too.

Help yourself to help your child

We wanted to use this chapter to think about how parents can help their children, through helping themselves. We realize that not everything discussed in this chapter will be relevant for everyone, but the ideas are important ones to think about. We will start by thinking about what we call 'vicarious learning', and how children learn from us as parents without us even realizing at times. We will then look at how making small behavioural changes ourselves can help children with anxiety, and how best to model these changes. Finally, we will discuss how you can best look after yourself and give you some strategies to help with this. Looking after yourself is so important – keeping healthy both physically and mentally as a parent can have such a positive impact on your children. Please keep at the forefront of your mind the idea that you must look after yourself first before you can look after others. While this is important in all situations, it is especially important when there are extra stresses within the family and you have to find extra energy and resilience to manage daily life.

Vicarious learning

Being a parent is a difficult job; there is no rule book and no one to tell you how to do things better. It is challenging and tiring. Despite all these difficulties, it can also be one of the most rewarding experiences. There is nothing that we wouldn't do for our children to ensure they have happy and healthy lives. At the same time, children learn so much from us as parents. They watch us to learn how to respond to certain situations, or how to 'do' certain behaviours, or perform particular chores. Children are soaking up information from us, like sponges, watching and learning from the environment around them.

As parents, perhaps we don't always realize how much children learn and copy us. Usually it is only noticeable when our children say something they shouldn't, and we notice that they have learned it from us. However, children do learn many things from us, including how we manage our own emotions and how we manage our own lives.

Vicarious learning happens when a child learns through watching a parent's behaviour without them offering direct instruction or teaching. For example, if a parent screams and runs away each time they see a spider, the child will learn that spiders are scary and is likely to react in the same way. The child will not have been directly taught that spiders are scary, but will have learned this from watching how their parents behave around spiders. Children learn about other emotions from parents, too. If a parent has anxiety in any area of their life, it is likely the child will be anxious in some way, too. Rosenbaum et al. (2000) looked at how many children of parents with panic disorder and depression had difficulties themselves. They found that there was a significant link between those parents who had panic disorder and depression and the likelihood of them having children who would demonstrate some similar symptoms, with behaviours being noticeable before the age of six years.

While no one can help having anxiety or depression, seeking help for it is important. It is important for your child to not vicariously learn some of the behaviours and symptoms of anxiety, and also important for your child to see you as a parent, seeking help – they need to understand that this okay to do. Anxiety and depression are treatable and manageable, and it is important for children to see their parents trying to help themselves. The information about managing anxiety difficulties in this book, while written to help children, is based on general principles, and the interventions included here can be used by adults, too. A parent showing any positive change in managing a situation differently will have a positive impact on a child through vicarious learning.

Behavioural changes and modelling

Behavioural changes are the one thing we have control over, and they can make such a difference to the way we manage the world and some of the challenges within it. Making simple changes can have a positive effect on our own wellbeing and that of our children. In Chapter 1 there is a discussion about reassurance: it is worth reading this again, as reassurance is one of the behaviours that will be relevant to all anxiety disorders and therefore to all children and parents. Knowing how to manage reassurance is so important, especially when it comes to shifting the responsibility back on to your child, to help them develop confidence and independence in being able to reassure themselves.

Looking after yourself through simple behaviour changes is a good place to start; we all pick up bad habits through life rather than doing the things that we should. Below are some of the things that we can do to make positive behaviour changes every day:

Positive behaviour changes	
• Good diet.	• Spend time with others.
• Reduce caffeine.	• Prioritise 'me' time.
• Exercise.	• Reduce alcohol intake.
• Good sleep patterns.	• Do not smoke.

Demonstrating good patterns of behaviours helps your children learn from you. It will keep your own physical and mental wellbeing strong, and will give you more resilience in managing the challenging days. This is called 'modelling', as you are modelling how someone should behave to establish positive physical and mental wellbeing. Your child will see you modelling these behaviours and will learn from them.

Taking time for yourself is important and is something that many of us forget to do. It is sometimes the simple things that can impact the most. These basic behaviour changes are the foundations of resilient parenting. Resilience is needed for any parent, but when your child has anxiety, you will need extra strength and resilience, and it is in going back to the fundamentals of looking after yourself that will improve this. Figure 2.1 shows a parenting resilience triangle which shows you what you need to be able to do yourself in order to manage some of the challenges you are faced with, and to develop resilience in your children.

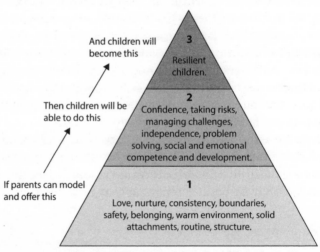

Figure 2.1 Pyramid of developing resilience in children

The benefits of self-care

Parenting can evoke within us many different feelings that can sometimes be surprisingly intense. When we are actively parenting and engaging with our child, these processes are naturally highly absorbing of our time and emotional resources – no matter how many moments of joy and enrichment we may experience. Being emotionally present and available for our child can be very challenging when there are other worries about health, relationships, finances, employment stability, losses or other changes in our circumstances. Add in other ingredients such as self-critical and judgemental thoughts, perfectionistic ideals or unrelenting standards (Young and Klosko, 1993) and parenting tasks might then become increasingly overwhelming, complex and challenging.

The concept of 'self-care' has gained a great deal of traction on social media, and for good reason: ensuring that we feel well in ourselves, as well as being tuned-in to our own needs and boundaries, gives us a good foundation to participate in life as well as the daily tasks of parenting.

What is self-care exactly, and is self-care enough?

As we described above, self-care can include taking an active role in daily tasks of living such as getting enough sleep and exercise, not over- or under-doing it by eating too much or too little of certain foods, not drinking too much alcohol, participating in activities that give us a sense of purpose or joy, keeping ourselves clean, and attending necessary health appointments. Making these behavioural changes and caring for ourselves becomes especially important when we are faced with increased pressures and stressful circumstances. Nevertheless, it is often quite tricky for us to implement these changes for a number of reasons. Unhelpful behaviours may be very familiar to us as we have been practising them for a long time; we might struggle with our motivation to make the behavioural changes needed, or perhaps struggle to keep these changes going (Riegel, Dunbar, Fitzsimons, et al. 2019).

Engaging in self-care (or even beginning to think about the idea of looking after ourselves) can sometimes bring up strong thoughts and beliefs about ourselves or ideas about parenting. These beliefs and perceptions are frequently influenced by our own experiences of being parented or watching others parent. When trying to support families and parents, parents often say that they don't have any time for self-care, they may not feel that they are worthy, or that self-care is not possible or worthwhile, or that it just isn't appealing to put their emotional and physical health before that of their children.

Thinking of our own needs and putting these first can feel uncomfortable, selfish and shameful, particularly if our own child is struggling with worries and anxiety that we feel take priority.

Sometimes, the worries we have about others can unintentionally distract us from our own difficult experiences or personal worries. These psychological barriers and obstacles are not to be underestimated or minimized; it often takes considerable courage for parents to acknowledge them, and to do the emotional work that is required in order for them to accept and care for themselves.

Similarly, you might find that giving yourself permission to take time out to focus and nurture yourself when you are used to looking after everyone else might feel like visiting a strange and unfamiliar country. It might feel uncomfortable or self-indulgent. If you feel you are able and willing to be open to new ways of thinking about and responding to yourself, doing so will likely lead to positive changes in your own and others' levels of well-being, and strengthen your ability to manage emotions and get through the stressful times in life. Ultimately, if we can nurture ourselves, we will be in a better place to be able to take care of the needs of our children.

Taking care of ourselves

There are a number of things we can do to change the ways in which we look after ourselves. It can be helpful to make some time to sit and think about what might help or challenge us when trying to make things feel better for ourselves.

The following worksheets present some questions you can ask yourself. Writing down clearly what helps you can be really useful.

Worksheet 1: Feeling emotionally connected

Work through the following questions. Be specific about the activities or things that you feel are helpful such as 'going for a walk in my local (name of place) park', 'watching birds in my garden in the morning', 'smelling vanilla pods', or naming a specific music track you like to listen to, rather than more generic ideas such as 'exercise', 'music' and so on.

What helps me feel emotionally well?
e.g. activities, time alone, healthy relationships, hobbies, paying attention to how we are feeling and responding compassionately, setting boundaries and saying 'no' etc.

What helps me feel physically well?
e.g. sleep, exercise, diet, routines, having a massage etc.

What makes me feel soothed?
e.g. nice smells and aromas, fluffy textures, giving myself a hug or wrapping a blanket around snugly, a warm bath, handcream or lotions, being in natural environments, looking at pictures of nature, music, warm drinks etc.

What makes me feel comforted?
e.g. acknowledging any tricky feelings and responding to myself in a kind and self-compassionate way, imagining what my best friend might say, watching a comforting movie or ambient screen saver, listening to comforting sounds (rain, the sea etc.), thinking of things that bring a sense of gratitude, spirituality etc.

What makes me feel connected to others?
e.g. what activities bring a sense of connectedness and purpose? work, hobbies, voluntary work, being with friends, increased eye contact, being in the moment, trust, making time to be with others, really listening to others with empathy etc.

Worksheet 2: Managing challenges and developing opportunities

It can also be helpful to try and imagine the obstacles and barriers, and situations that can get in the way of you being able to look after yourself. Work through the following questions to try and identify any challenges you are facing, and to identify opportunities you can develop.

What might get in the way of me looking after myself? (practically or psychologically)
e.g. not putting time in the diary or calendar, putting in too many other activities, not knowing when or where to start, other adults invalidating my needs, feeling self-care is a weakness, feeling guilty or unworthy, feeling unmotivated etc.

What might make it harder to look after myself?
e.g. being a single parent, little social support, working long hours, family sickness or ill-health, feeling mentally unwell such as being low in mood or very anxious etc.

What might help me to overcome these challenges to look after myself?
e.g. giving myself permission to take care of me, making time to explore what makes me feel soothed, comforted or connected, asking others for help, strengthening social relationships, learning to plan my time, doing something I know I like even if I don't feel in the mood, getting professional therapeutic support if feeling mentally unwell etc.

When we feel more able to nurture and care for ourselves with kindness and compassion, we may find we have more emotional space, tolerance and patience to deal with the emotions and behavioural challenges that our children need our help and support with. Developing our abilities to soothe and comfort ourselves when we are feeling calm will put us in a strong position to respond helpfully – by first calming down our own reactions and responses to our child's emotions and behaviours before then attending to our child's behaviours and any hidden emotional needs.

Summary

Understanding the impact you have on your child, in terms of their vicarious learning and the way you model behaviours, is key to helping your child learn positively from you. However, you must ensure that you look after yourself to be a positive role model and manage the stresses of daily parenting life with a child who has anxiety.

By using the forms in this chapter to develop a list of ways in which you can use self-care, and manage some of the challenges associated with this, you will ensure that you are in the best possible state of mind to help your child.

References and further reading

Riegel, B., Dunbar, S.B., Fitzsimons, D., Freedland, K.E., Lee, C.S., Middleton, S., Stromberg, A., Vellone, E., Webber, D.E. and Jaarsma, T. (2019) 'Self-care research: Where are we now? Where are we going?' *Int. J. Nurs. Stud.* 103402.

Rosenbaum et al., (2000) 'Controlled Study of Behavioral Inhibition in Children of Parents with Panic Disorder and Depression', *American Journal of Psychiatry*, 157(12), pp.2002–2010.

Young, J.E. and Klosko, J.S. (1993) *Reinventing Your Life: How to Break Free From Negative Life Patterns*. New York: Dutton.

3
Common fears and phobias

Sam Thompson, RMN & CBT Therapist

This chapter will look at common fears and phobias. We will first look at how common fears are described by, and present in, children. We'll also look at some of the most common phobias, such as fear of spiders, fear of being sick or fear of going to school. The chapter then offers some strategies for overcoming these fears.

A phobia can often be described as an incredibly strong and persistent fear, which is caused by being exposed to a certain situation or object. Fears and phobias are relatively common and are experienced by people of all ages. Adults can experience a variety of phobias, ranging from haemophobia (the fear of blood) to aviophobia (the fear of flying). These fears and worries can have a significant impact on a person's well-being, as well as their ability to manage in the given situation. People with such fears will 'overestimate' the actual threat from the situation or object (see Chapter 11). They may also describe themselves as 'overthinkers', experiencing several thoughts at once when feeling anxious.

Children's fears may transfer in different ways, many of which we may not expect to typically see. Common fears and phobias among children include arachnophobia (fear of spiders), emetophobia (fear of being sick) and social phobia (fear of being in a social environment). Social phobia tends to be a bit trickier, but we will explore this in further detail in Chapter 7. The next section describes common phobias in more detail and offers various strategies that you can use to support your children.

Arachnophobia (fear of spiders)

Spider phobias are one of many common anxiety disorders, and have an impact on between 3.5–6.1 per cent of the general population. When people are faced with a spider, they experience an intense sense of fear and a reluctance to look at it any further (Leutgeb, Schäfer and Schienle, 2009). This fearful feeling leads to an increase in avoidance behaviours, whereby people will go to great lengths to not be exposed to this phobia (see Chapter 1, Figure 1.5). For example, someone with arachnophobia may avoid entering certain parts of the house where they've previously encountered a spider. Having asked someone to remove the spider on their behalf, they will be reluctant to enter the same room again. As with all phobias, the continued reluctance to see the initial source of the fear increases the levels of distress and upset for people. Your child may have a tendency to become increasingly worried or upset when being asked to do everyday tasks, or during their bedtime routine.

Emetophobia (fear of being sick)

Emetophobia is often described as the intense fear that a young person has around feeling or thinking that they are going to be sick (Veale, 2009). A child experiencing emetophobia may feel incredibly worried about being sick in front of other people. They may have different perceptions around food and what they can or can't eat. For example, your child may choose not to eat junk food or dairy produce because they worry that this would make them feel sick. Being sick in front of people is often one of a child's greatest fears. They are worried about the negative response and reaction to the situation and will try to do as much as they can to prevent such a thing from happening. Children may feel incredibly reluctant to eat out in restaurants or other public places. A child with emetophobia may also feel repulsed by witnessing others feeling, or indeed being, sick. This fear can stay with a child for a considerable amount of time, unless there has been a suitable intervention.

Emetophobia is often traced to early childhood where, typically, there will have been a traumatic experience relating to feeling sick, being sick or observing a situation involving sickness. Your child may be able to recall the moment or moments when their emetophobia started to develop. However, don't assume that your child can immediately recall when they began to feel higher levels of anxiety with the emetophobia. Children who experience emetophobia often describe the feeling that they are going to be sick but this correlates to the feeling of anxiety and these symptoms tend to overlap, especially in relation to the phobia. These symptoms are ever present and often the catalyst for an overwhelming feeling of anxiety. Peculiar eating habits and restriction of dietary intake can often be misdiagnosed for an eating disorder or eating related difficulties.

If your child is experiencing emetophobia, then it is common for them to also experience social phobia (see Chapter 7). At that point it becomes difficult to separate and distinguish between both aspects, especially as eating or going out in public can often make young people feel sick.

School phobia

School phobia refers to a child's initial refusal to want to attend school. There is often a tendency for children to display behaviours associated with not wanting to attend school, such as feeling angry and frustrated. Children may also become distressed and upset, as well as showing signs of worry when it comes to attending school. These behaviours may be more common the night before the start of the school week, or returning after a school holiday. Children may also describe some physical symptoms relating to worry, such as complaining that they feel sick, or in some cases, may be sick due to their anxiety.

There is a tendency for a child experiencing school phobia to continue experiencing further worries, especially if they are spending prolonged periods away from their educational environment. They may begin to feel worried about being unable to catch up on school work, missing the interaction with their school friends and due to these and potentially other factors may be more reluctant in wanting to return to school.

It is important to acknowledge and recognize that there is a significant difference between school refusal and truancy. Truancy is often associated with antisocial behaviour, rather than emotional upset, and parents tend to be unaware that it is happening. It is important to raise the young person's difficulties in attending school with the appropriate contact at their school.

It is also common to see children being moved to a different school as parents hope it will provide a solution to their children's difficulties. However, for a child who has school phobia, a change in environment is really just a temporary fix, like putting a sticking plaster on a broken bone. It is important to recognize your best efforts as a parent, especially when trying to support your child and find the most appropriate solution. We also understand that as a parent you do not want your child to have difficulties with attending school, but applying various strategies and skills can help them overcome their worries and be able to reintegrate back into a school environment once again. If you have any concerns about school attendance and would like further support then make sure you contact your child's school support team or appropriate Children's Adolescent Mental Health Service (CAMHS). As with emetophobia, school phobia may often be related to social phobia (see Chapter 7 for more information).

Approaches to phobias

Avoiding the fear

We often hear about the term 'avoidance', especially in the context of procrastination and a reluctance to participate in an activity, but how does avoidance impact on a young person with a specific phobia or fear of a situation? Avoidance can have a detrimental impact on their fear. For example, since we often see spiders in the garden (especially under rocks), your child may be reluctant to go outside, even if the weather is warm and it is summer. A child often cannot express what they are thinking at that moment in time, so you might see a change in behaviour or emotions first hand. Here's an example:

Billy
Billy is seven years old and lives with his mum and dad, as well as his older sister who is ten years old. Billy has often been described by his parents as a 'worrier', ever since he was little. Mum and Dad report that Billy has a fear of spiders which has developed signifi-cantly over the last year or so when he saw a 'big' spider crawl out

from under a rock in the garden. Ever since then, Billy has not been in the garden. Even in the summer, Billy will choose to stay inside while his family have barbecues and sit in the garden. Billy is now unwilling to use the bathroom downstairs because he knows that spiders will be in there.

The example above demonstrates how Billy's stressful encounter with spiders has caused him to feel increasingly worried whenever he is in a situation that has the potential to include spiders. Billy's worry continues to increase, and he is continuing to try to avoid any encounter with spiders due to his fear of seeing one. As we saw in Chapter 1, avoiding situations can increase the level of worry and distress – it's important to reflect that back to young people, especially with the impact avoidance can have on worry.

Be curious

If your child is currently experiencing a phobia then it can be incredibly distressing and upsetting for both themselves and the rest of your family. Younger children may be blissfully unaware of what's happening, but they are incredibly susceptible to understanding distress and upset from their siblings (see 'vicarious learning' in Chapter 2). It is important to leave the emotions 'at the door', especially with how you are feeling as a parent. For someone experiencing a phobia, if it was that simple to treat then no one would develop them. Instead, adopt a curious approach to your questions, especially when talking to children. Often, we use the analogy of an old-fashioned detective with a magnifying glass, searching for clues. We need to know why the child is feeling upset or angry. For example, you could say:

> 'Can you tell me how you're feeling?'
> 'What's happening?'
> 'I've noticed you've been feeling upset about attending school. Can you talk to me about what's going on?'

It's important to adopt a curious, inquisitive approach toward a child, especially if they're feeling worried about not attending school.

Offering 'open' questions (questions that cannot be answered with 'yes' or 'no') can help to encourage children to talk about their worries without the fear of being judged. It is often the case in children that they may have worries about getting into trouble.

Reassurance

For parents and staff working in educational settings, we may find that it can be an automatic response to want to reassure the young person. As human beings, we do not like to see them upset and distressed, so we attempt to reassure them to improve the situation. For a child with a phobia, however, a constant theme of reassurance or reassurance-seeking behaviour will reiterate to them that they cannot cope with what is going on. As phobia treatment involves prolonged exposure to a feared object or situation, the time spent feeling uncomfortable will mean that they will attempt to avoid what they are afraid of. Try to avoid reassuring your child too much; although it is tempting to reassure them constantly, it won't help them manage the problem. In fact, it might even increase their tendency to avoid situations. This is because high levels of reassurance from someone does not provide a long-term solution to the difficulties they are experiencing. It can also increase the levels of 'safety behaviours' where children continue to avoid certain situations.

In this conversation, the parent is giving only minimal reassurance:

Parent: Rosie, I noticed that recently you've not been wanting to go to school. What's been going on?

Rosie: I don't want to talk about it.

Parent: I understand that you don't want to talk about it at the moment but I'm here for you if you want to talk. I've noticed that you've been very sad recently and I'm not sure what's happening. Have you been feeling sad?

Rosie: Sometimes I feel sad.

Parent: Okay, so you feel sad. I can see that from the expression on your face. Is there anything that you're feeling? You usually like school, don't you?

Rosie: School makes me feel sad.

Parent: Why does school make you feel sad?

Rosie: Well, I don't like it. People are mean to me.

The example above shows how adopting a curious approach with children can encourage them to talk about how they're feeling, and explain what's going on for them at that moment in time. It is important to not show any forms of overreaction or any potential anger or fear to the child, as they can process this information differently. With children, the use of emojis can work well, especially if they aren't sure about what they're feeling. Children can be excellent in recognizing emojis and different facial expressions. You can purchase emoji dice from various places (see Further Resources). There's also no right or wrong answer when it comes to guessing the emojis as young people will interpret feelings differently to others. To correct a child may come across as invalidating or rejecting their feelings.

Ladder (exposure to the fear)

For children who are experiencing any form of phobia, the thought of confronting it is quite simply terrifying. If you put it into perspective, if there is something that you have wanted to put off for such a long time, then you are asked to confront the fear in question, it is going to make you feel incredibly uncomfortable. One of the ways to help children overcome their fears and worries in relation to their phobia is to develop a ladder of exposure. We place the least feared object or situation at the bottom, and work up the rungs of the ladder together, in a collaborative effort. It's important to highlight the collaboration as it will be more meaningful to the child and they will be more likely to want to do it. Figure 3.1 shows an example of a ladder for a young person who has emetophobia:

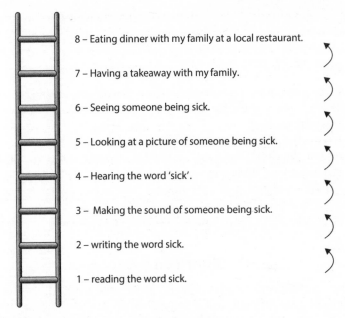

Figure 3.1 Example of an exposure ladder

Using an exposure ladder ensures that your child isn't overwhelmed by a prolonged exposure to their phobia.

Too much fear is called 'flooding' and this might leave your child feeling more traumatized in the future. A collaborative exposure ladder instead can help your child to identify what they need to do to overcome the fear. This is because when someone experiences worry or fear, subconsciously they are being told that they cannot do it, and that it is dangerous, as this is what the threat system is ringing the alarm bell for. Small, gradual steps on the ladder can instil confidence in your child. If you have any doubts about building and using an 'exposure ladder' with your child, speak to a CAMHS worker or suitable clinician.

Reluctance to ask for help

Children who are experiencing phobias may also be reluctant to seek help and support to help overcome this. Your child might find it hard to talk about what is going on and they may have perceptions that fearful events would happen if they did. It is important to encourage children to develop the skills that they need to overcome their fears or worries. Further support can be found through your local CAMHS service and through the resources at the end of this chapter. Here is an example of how a conversation may play out:

> **Parent**: Jeremiah, I know you've been having some difficulty with eating meals over the last few weeks. Is everything okay? You used to enjoy my cooking.
> **Jeremiah**: I don't want to eat anything at the moment.
> **Parent**: Why not? You usually do! How do you feel when at mealtimes?
> **Jeremiah**: I feel really nervous and worried about what I'm eating.
> **Parent**: I understand your feelings but I'm interested to know what it is you're nervous about?
> **Jeremiah**: Well, I feel sick when I eat, and I don't want to eat, really.

Distraction skills

When a child is feeling particularly anxious or worried, they may often find it difficult to articulate their thoughts. Depending on the severity of the anxiety that the child is experiencing, they may continue to become increasingly anxious. If exposure to the situation is accelerating this for your child, then you can encourage them to use distraction to reduce their worry. Distraction can be effective in helping the young person not to think about what is causing them this level of distress. All children have their own unique set of distraction skills: speak to them about what might help them relax if they're feeling worried. You can call it a toolkit or something similar, and encourage them to decorate it with what they like doing. Below are some examples of what a distraction kit may contain:

Distraction kit examples

- Draw a picture.
- Make slime.
- Use a fidget toy.
- Play on a table.
- Talk to friends/family.

Emoji time

Many children find it hard to distinguish between what thoughts and feelings actually are. It is easy to become confused as they have a tendency to overlap when talking about how they're thinking and feeling. It's important to break down what it is they're actually feeling. Often you may notice certain behaviours, such as handwashing for example, or that they become highly anxious about a situation that they're fearful of. Recognizing and understanding emotions can help children to understand how they're feeling. With younger children, the use of emojis can help them understand their feelings if they're reluctant to talk at that time. Figure 3.3 shows some emojis that have been made to describe common emotions that people may experience. Try this exercise in exploring feelings:

1 Print out the emoji list in Figure 3.2 (or similar).
2 Cut out each emoji.
3 Place the emojis in a bowl.
4 Ask your child to pick out an emoji and explain what it means to them.

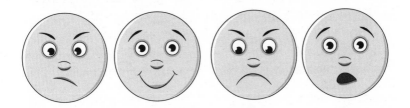

Figure 3.2 Emoji list

The conversation might go as follows:

Adult: In this bowl, I've got a handful of different emojis. Now, I don't really use emojis, so I what I would like you to do is to take out each one and tell me what you think what emotion each emoji represents. Does that make sense?

Aayan: Yes!

Aayan picks out 'worried' emoji from the bowl

Adult: What emoji is that?

Aayan: It looks like 'worried' or 'scared', I think.

Adult: What makes you say that, Aayan?

Aayan: The mouth is like a zig-zag, which often means that you're worried about something.

Adult: What makes you feel worried?

Aayan: Lots of things. I worry that my family will get hurt or kidnapped.

It's important not to guess the emojis for your child, and to give the time for them to work out what they are. They may need some prompting with working out and understanding certain emojis. This is a particularly effective method when using electronic devices, such as tablets and smartphones.

Writing it down

When children are feeling particularly anxious or worried about a certain situation they often tend to ruminate about their thoughts or feelings. Although we are not mind readers and don't claim to be, we can see certain ways in which children may act, especially when experiencing obsessions and compulsions. One way to help manage this is to encourage children to write down the worries they're experiencing in a table similar to the one below. The table encourages children to externalize their experiences when they've felt particularly worried. Each column breaks down the current situation into what was happening, as well as their thoughts and feelings.

What was going on?	How it made me feel	What I was thinking about	What I did
Didn't want to go back to school after the weekend.	Initially felt worried and stressed but relieved afterwards.	I don't like school, I feel that no one likes me. The work is too hard.	I went to talk to my Mum about it.

Figure 3.3 Example of a worry table example

A common metaphor to help children understand and explore their emotions is the use of the 'iceberg'. You can explain what an iceberg is and what it looks like. Encourage your child to draw one if it helps to aid their understanding. Reflect back to the young person what it is they've drawn:

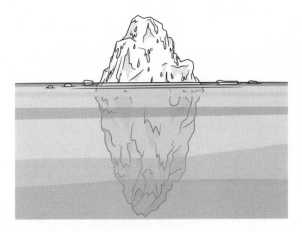

Figure 3.4 Iceberg conversation example

Parent: So, Carin, can you tell me what you've drawn?

Carin: It's an iceberg.

Parent: Excellent, that's a great looking iceberg! Do you know what an iceberg is?

Carin: It's something in the sea. I remember learning about the *Titanic* in school.

Parent: Oh really? What happened to the *Titanic*?

Carin: The *Titanic* hit the iceberg.

Parent: It did! Well remembered. What is it about icebergs that are unusual?

Carin: You can only see the tip of the iceberg.

Parent: You can, that's correct. Do you know what's underneath? Are you able to draw it for me?

Carin: Yeah, I think so.

Parent: So what we can see is the top part, can't we? We don't see what's underneath. Sometimes what can happen is that people may see us feeling scared or angry but they don't know what else we're feeling. Like with the iceberg, they don't see what's underneath. Does that make sense?

Carin: Yeah it does.

Parent: And how does that relate to how you feel, Carin?
Carin: When I feel angry, I also feel scared and confused but no one else sees that.

Summary

This chapter has offered a range of strategies for children who may be experiencing fears or phobias. Phobias are common to all of us. Having a clear plan, using a ladder hierarchy, and being curious about why our children feel the way they do, can help overcome these difficulties. Many of the strategies discussed in this chapter give you and your child opportunity to have fun and be creative in managing their anxieties while in fact spending quality time together.

References and further reading

Leutgeb, V., Schäfer, A. and Schienle, A. (2009) 'An event-related potential study on exposure therapy for patients suffering from spider phobia', *Biological Psychology*, 82(3), pp.293–300.

Öst, L.G., Salkovskis, P.M. and Hellström, K. (1991) 'One-session therapist-directed exposure vs. self-exposure in the treatment of spider phobia', *Behavior Therapy*, 22(3), pp.407–422.

Veale, D. (2009) 'Cognitive behaviour therapy for a specific phobia of vomiting', *Cognitive Behaviour Therapist*, 2(4).

Online resources

Anxiety UK. *Free anxiety resources.* <www.anxietyuk.org.uk/get-help/free-anxiety-resources/>

Barnardos. *What is anxiety?* <www.barnardos.org.uk/blog/what-anxiety>

Learning Resources. *Emoji Cubes* <www.learningresources.co.uk/emoji-cubes>

MindEd. *MindEd Hub.* <www.minded.org.uk>

NHS. *Anxiety in children.* <www.nhs.uk/conditions/stress-anxiety-depression/anxiety-in-children/>

NHS. *NHS Apps Library.* <www.nhs.uk/apps-library/>

NHS. *Looking after a child or young person's mental health.* <www.nhs.uk/oneyou/every-mind-matters/childrens-mental-health/>

Stem4. *Anxiety for teenagers.* <stem4.org.uk/anxiety/anxiety-for-teenagers/>

The Working Together Team. *Might Moe: An Anxiety Workbook for Children.*
<website.twtt.org.uk/media/Mighty%20Moe1%20Anxiety.pdf>
Young Minds. *Anxiety.* <youngminds.org.uk/find-help/conditions/anxiety/>
YoungMinds (2020) *Parents Guide To Support – School Anxiety And Refusal.*
<youngminds.org.uk/find-help/for-parents/parents-guide-to-support-
a-z/#school-anxiety-and-refusal>

4

Generalized worries and anxieties

Ann Cox, RMN & CBT Therapist
Ben Lea, RMN & CBT Therapist

This chapter looks at generalized worries and anxieties. Generalized worries are not related to other types of distinct worries, such as phobias, or worries about school or something bad that has happened, as discussed in other chapters in this book. Generalized worries are best described as the 'what if' worries, and are usually future orientated. These worries can be about anything and can become very troublesome for your child. Sometimes these worries are related to things happening in your child's life, other times they can be about existential (life and death) events, such as planets colliding or natural disasters (including famines and other catastrophic, although unlikely, events). This chapter will give you a detailed overview of generalized worries and will also provide you with a wide range of strategies that you and your child can try to alleviate some of the symptoms.

What is generalized worry?

Generalized worry is very common in children and adolescents, and current estimates suggest that anywhere between 8–22 per cent of children and adolescents may suffer from an anxiety disorder (NHS Digital, 2020). We also know that difficulties surrounding generalized worry are most likely to start between the ages of 11 and the early 20s and is more common in females, although generalized worry in younger children is not unusual.

Although anxiety is very common in children, there are many different types of anxiety. Some children might struggle with specific phobias, such as becoming extremely anxious when a dog is present; others might struggle with social situations, and others might feel anxious when they experience perceived physical health problems.

The difference with someone who struggles with generalized worry is that they may experience some of the anxieties of the social phobic or health worrier, but they are not specific to this area, they are generalized. In a similar fashion, children can worry about various other future-based aspects of life and situations, while also worrying about possible outcomes of their worries in the future ('worrying about worries').

A good way to describe a generalized worrier would be a child who worries about the many aspects of life that are difficult for them to control. The child may be seen as a 'worrier' by others; they may appear overly cautious and may often seek reassurances from others, while avoiding particular situations due to fears of something bad happening. A child with these types of worries may also feel that worrying is a good thing, it keeps them safe. Worrying allows them to stop 'bad' things from happening and allows them to prepare if anything 'bad' was to take place. Although adults might identify with this, and agree that worrying can be helpful, it can become a significant problem for a child. A child worrying about lots of things that are very unlikely to happen right now (such as death, or not having enough time to complete something, or planets colliding and so on), may stop doing activities they would normally enjoy if they weren't worrying so much.

What are the symptoms and what might a parent see?

Symptoms in generalized worriers might look a little different when compared to other anxieties. Children who constantly worry about various future-related situations will always have some level of anxiety 'bubbling' – this may not be particularly severe. A child who is scared of dogs and comes into contact with one, or a child with social anxiety who has been asked to read out in front of their class, would experience much more severe symptom distress. With 'bubbling' generalized worries, the levels of extreme anxiety may be less evident but they are present for long periods of time. In generalized worry, there might not always be clear triggers for a child's anxiety that a parent can identify.

The initial step in helping your child to overcome anxiety is to recognize it, but this can be difficult. Children struggling with generalized worries can be cautious and shy; some may be very eager to please and comply with others around them. However, some anxious children may also present differently, with challenging behaviours that could include tantrums or disobedience. Anyone observing these behaviours may conclude that the child is simply naughty, not that they are incredibly anxious. The iceberg analogy in Chapter 3 is a great way to think more about a child's behaviour; sometimes there can be more than meets the eye when a child is acting in a particular way. Any behaviour is a form of communication, and framing behaviour in this way can be helpful as you explore what the child is trying to communicate.

Symptoms that might be seen in a generalized worrier include:

- Reassurance seeking – this might be verbal reassurance, (for older children) text messages, reassurance from friends or from the internet.
- Distracted.
- Restlessness or feeling on edge.
- Easily fatigued.
- Muscle tension.
- Difficulties in concentrating.
- Problems with sleeping (getting to sleep and staying asleep).
- Irritability.

These symptoms can understandably be difficult to spot at times, as they can overlap with many other difficulties that might be present. Someone struggling with obsessive thoughts might seek reassurance as a result of these thoughts and someone who is very low in mood and stressed might present as tense, fatigued and struggling with their concentration. Common symptoms are seen across many difficulties, determining their cause is important, as this will inform the support your child needs.

To help with thinking about these symptoms, it can be useful to think a little more broadly in terms of when and why these symptoms are present. For more help with this, I would recommend reading the section on 'talking to your child' in Chapter 7. This will help you think more about when your child's difficulty becomes a problem, where it's a problem, and in which situation(s) it might be present.

Impact of generalized worrying

There are many ways in which generalized worrying can impact on a child. It is helpful to think about a child in their three main environments: home, school and social. By recognizing some of these impacts, you'll be able to identify if your child is struggling with generalized worry. These impacts are not particular to generalized worries and can be seen in other forms of anxiety – finding out the cause of the impact, or symptom, is important to ensure the right support and help is given to your child.

Personal impacts

On a personal level for your child, worry can reduce confidence. You may see changes in your child in a reduction of what they used to be able to do in comparison to what they do now: they might stop doing a hobby they used to do, or certain activities. Children who worry more may spend less time with their friends, spend more time in their bedroom and may be seeking more reassurance from a parent or close family member or friend. High levels of anxiety are also associated with low mood. Low mood impacts on motivation and concentration, and your child can become more negative and more self-critical with reduced self-esteem. If you add the continuous worries themselves to these symptoms you can see how debilitating generalized worry can be. Your child may be distracted and have reduced concentration. They may struggle to get off to sleep. Worries seem to be more prevalent at night, so keeping a check on how your child is sleeping will be helpful to understand the full scope of the impact of their worries.

What strategies can you use to support the personal impacts?

When children start to withdraw or do less than they did before, getting them to restart things and be around people more is really helpful. The anxiety cycle can be a bit of a vicious circle. Figure 4.1 shows this vicious circle for generalized worries:

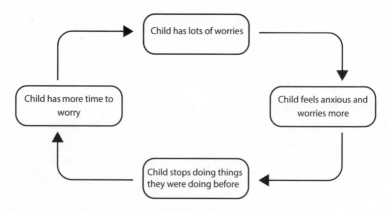

Figure 4.1 Vicious circle for generalized worries

Trying to reverse some of the things that your child has stopped doing will give them less time for thinking about worries, and will get them engaged in more activities and with more people. What we know about low mood, which comes hand in hand with anxiety, is that the more physical activity and the more connection we have with other people, the better our mood. You can help by getting your child to spend more time out of their room, doing family activities and supporting them to spend more time with their friends or connecting with nature, which has proven positive effects on increasing mood and reducing anxiety (see Chapter 1). If you are able to improve your child's mood, then this will have a positive effect on their anxiety.

Self-criticism can be common in generalized worriers and those with a low mood. Self-criticism from a child can be hard to hear, especially when you can see clearly that it is not true. However, telling a child it is not true when they are feeling like this can be unhelpful. Your child might feel like you are not understanding or validating how they are feeling. Helping your child to see things more objectively in a positive way can help. Writing down three good or positive things that have happened each day can be helpful for your child, giving them a short break from the negativity. Looking for positive things in opportune moments will slowly break the cycle of negativity, especially when it is linked with more activity. This could be naming what a good time you have had, or verbalizing how much you enjoyed that cup of tea. Small, positive affirmations can be really helpful in breaking the cycle of negativity and self-criticism.

Impacts on home life

Seeking continual reassurance from parents or any care giver is probably the most impactful aspect of worry within the home. It is normal for you as a parent to reassure your child, but there is a point where reassurance can become unhelpful. We looked at this in Chapter 1 and offered strategies that can be used to help your child reassure themselves. Having worry can make your child more dependent on you, and seeking reassurance is one such typical behaviour. Helping your child to become more independent is really good for challenging worries. It will reduce the reassurance-seeking and it will increase your child's self-confidence. If your child can reassure themselves, they will have developed a really good skill that they can take with them through to adulthood.

Your child may also seem to regress, meaning that they may act as if they were younger than their chronological years. This is a common occurrence in children. A child may do this if they feel psychologically unsafe. All the worries and symptoms they have are causing them high levels of anxiety. By acting like a younger child, the child is trying to get parents to offer a more intensive level of support. We have seen how behaviour is a form of communication, and this is a typical example.

What strategies can you use to support the impacts at home?

We discussed reassurance in Chapter 1, so return to this for some helpful ideas about helping yourself to not reassure your child more than what is usual, and supporting your child to reassure themselves. If your child learns how to reassure themselves, they are developing independence and this will in turn increase their general confidence in managing certain situations and worries. This will also improve their mood and have a positive impact on their ability to manage their anxiety. Improving independence in a child is really easy and can be done in so many ways, for example:

- Using tools: scissors, knives, woodwork or gardening tools.
- Responsibility: running errands, feeding the animals, laying the table, changing the bed.
- Increase their role in day-to-day activities: help make a meal, help with the gardening, help with the shopping.

Any of these activities will help to increase independence. By encouraging your child to further increase their independence in the activity each time they undertake it, you will be supporting your child to learn and grow at the same time. For example, if they are making a meal, on the first occasion you may help them with some of the tasks involved. If you're having crusty bread with the meal, on the first occasion you cut the bread, and your child butters it. On the second occasion, you support your child to cut the bread and they butter it. On the third occasion, your child cuts the bread independently and butters it by themselves. Although these strategies are not managing the anxiety directly, the increase in confidence and independence that come with them will have a positive effect in managing anxiety. The quality time that you and your child spend connecting with each other during these activities will also indirectly improve the anxiety and the worries that they have.

Impacts on school

When a child is worrying a lot about the 'what ifs', it can leave very little space in their heads for anything else. As a result, they might be very distracted in school. The understanding of what is required of them in class is not always fully taken in by a child who is distracted by worry. This can impact on their classwork and also their understanding of homework tasks. We know that children who have generalized worries can withdraw and don't want to be around other people, so if a teacher has noticed a change in your child's friendships or that they are spending more time alone, this could be an indicator that something is not quite right. Should the impacts within school not be picked up fairly quickly then there is a possibility of school becoming too overwhelming for your child, and they may start trying to take days off or miss certain lessons. If they start becoming more worried about school specifically, then it may be that the anxiety is sneaking into another difficulty such as social anxiety (which includes performance anxiety); your child may be worried about exams or talking out loud in class (Chapter 7); or your child may start with specific anxiety about attending school and develop a school phobia (Chapter 3). If this does happen, don't be alarmed by the fact that the anxiety is changing – it is very common with generalized worry for it to change and focus somewhere else. You will just need to refocus the strategies to be more specific about the cause of the anxiety, so in these instances, referring to the advice given in Chapters 3 and 7 will help.

What strategies can you use to support the impacts at school?

Your child can be helped by having information given to them verbally and also in written form. This will help with classwork and homework. Giving written and visual information at home will also be helpful. An example of this may be writing out a timetable, or providing a picture timetable of tasks for the day during the day; this may include meeting all of their hygiene needs, homework, chores, time for themselves. Other written information could include setting diary times for self-care, so the child can see this on a wall calendar or whiteboard to remind them. This gives your child the opportunity to go back and read the information when they are feeling less anxious. By having the written information, your child will feel more reassured. Schools should support you and your child by offering you a regular time each week to discuss any difficulties that are being experienced in school and look to see how they can help. Usually teachers who offer pastoral support will help and support children with such difficulties. It will be helpful for you to find out who these teachers are and make contact.

Keeping your child in a routine and attending school is helpful in managing anxiety in whatever form, as it keeps your child busy and distracted, more so than if they were sat at home in an unstructured environment. The more boundaries you can put around anxiety, the easier it is managed.

Impact on social life

We have already identified that withdrawal from social activities can impact on a child's life when they are struggling with generalized worries, and have explored strategies to improve this. Generalized worries can put strain on your child's friendships, often because your child is constantly worrying if they have done anything wrong within their friendships. The level of self-criticism your child has may make them feel that they are not worthy of being with their friends or that they are not good enough. When this occurs, it is likely that friendships will begin to dwindle.

Children's lives on social media can be another significant impact. They may be comparing themselves with others, leading to an increase in self-criticism. It is common for some children to publish self-deprecating information about themselves or publish how they are feeling as a way of reaching out for help – but this can leave the child extremely vulnerable to others' reactions. Children may forget or may not even be aware of the long-term consequences of posting information online and how this will remain in the ether forever, potentially causing difficulties for them later in life.

What strategies can you use to support the impacts in the social environment?

Speaking to your child about how they are managing their social media accounts may be a tricky subject to raise, but it is really important to have an open conversation. It is important that you know what your child is reading about, or publishing, on their accounts. By keeping an open dialogue with your child about social media, you will help them to stay safer online, reducing the potential for future difficulties while also reducing generalized worry. Internet matters (<www.internetmatters.org/>) is a great website that supports parents with this.

Keeping your child linked in with their friends, hobbies and social activities will also help. Keeping your child connected to their social environment will help prevent some of the potential withdrawal that anxiety and worries inevitably can cause. Connecting with nature helps in numerous ways, as we've said before. Get out of the house and go for that woodland walk; activity within nature is a great combination.

Strategies that can help with generalized worries

Keeping a routine and structure

We have discussed this briefly in the section about school and routine. Your child's generalized worries can increase when they are less busy and have more time to worry.

Controlling the worries rather than the worries controlling your child

If your child is able to set specific times for worrying, worry for the entire allocated time and then push other worries out of their head, they will take control of the worries rather than the worries controlling them. This is a hard thing to do. The 'worry time' should take place in an environment that is quite boring, not in their bedroom, living room or kitchen as these are safe and warm places in the house. We don't want to get anxious feelings mixed up with warm feelings. Places like utility rooms, garages, sheds or toilets can make great 'worry time' places.

Let's look at an example of worry time from Mohammed's day:

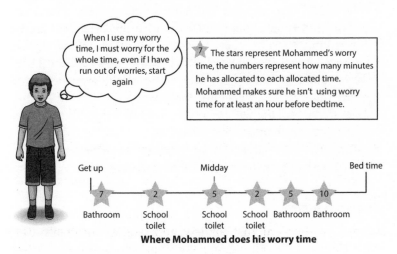

Where Mohammed does his worry time

Figure 4.2 An example of how to use worry time

The time allocated to each worry time is gauged on how much the child worries during that part of the day. Before you decide the time allocation, it is helpful if you and your child can try worrying for five minutes to see the challenges, then you can make an informed decision about what the time allocation should be. Once each week of worry time has been completed, changes can be made to the allocation of time. If it is working, then you can keep the same time or reduce it slightly. If it is not working, either more time or more allocations of time may be needed throughout the day. Ensuring that there is not a worry time allocated within an hour of going to bed will help your child to keep bedtime and nights worry-free. Worry time is difficult to do, but when it is done consistently and the full worry time allocation is used, then it can help your child gain control over their worries.

Refocusing your thoughts

1 By refocusing their thoughts your child can gain some control over what they are thinking in the present moment. Your child can do this in many ways, and you can have some fun with them. One easy way of doing this is by using the alphabet for a basis for topic discussions. Get your child to choose a topic they like – for example animals, sports people, characters, space and planets. Your child starts with the letter 'A', naming something, then 'B', then 'C' etc. For example, if the topic is animals, it may be Antelope, Beaver, Cow and so on, until they have found an animal for each letter of the alphabet going right through to 'Z' (Zebra). Refocussing and taking control over their thinking will help your child to feel more confident that they can manage their thoughts.
2 Another method that can be practised anywhere is the five senses technique which we provide in Chapter 12.

Bedtime routine

Having a nice, relaxing and structured bedtime routine can help with reducing generalized worries, especially if this is coupled with the worry time. At bedtime, activities that don't include any TV, iPads, games consoles or mobile phones or anything with *blue light* (the light emitted through technology), will help your child have a more peaceful sleep. Having a shower or bath before bed can help the body relax a little better. Activities such as reading, drawing or listening to music can also help to relax your child.

Summary

This chapter has included many strategies to help with generalized worries. Consistency is the key. Trying to manage scary or worrying thoughts is always going to be difficult, but perseverance will help to keep those worries under control.

Reference and further reading

NHS Digital (2020) *Mental Health of Children and Young People in England, 2020.* [Online]. Available at: <files.digital.nhs.uk/CB/C41981/mhcyp_2020_rep.pdf> (accessed: 25 October 2020).

5

Anxieties and neurodevelopmental conditions

Dr Laurence Baldwin, RMN

This chapter looks at how worries and anxieties show themselves in those with neurodevelopmental conditions, such as autism, ADHD, dyslexia and Tourette's (amongst others). Anxiety is very common among these young people, but is often not seen as such, because it shows itself in a number of ways that can be seen as negative behaviours. This chapter is about understanding how anxiety shows itself, and gives some ideas on how best to help.

What are neurodevelopmental conditions?

'Neurodevelopmental conditions' is a medical term used to describe a range of conditions that we are slowly getting better at understanding, and slowly the rest of the world is getting to understand. The term covers a wide range of different conditions, but most of them are obvious to people because of the behaviours that people with these conditions display. This has the big disadvantage that some people will think of these conditions mostly as being just those behaviours, rather than thinking about the person behind the behaviours, and what is causing those behaviours to happen.

Are labels useful?

The labels that are used to describe neurodevelopmental conditions are varied, and they reflect the history of how healthcare and medical professions have come to understand these conditions. The main ones (those with the largest number of people who have them) are ADHD and autism (ASD), but there are many more names for different types of neurodevelopmental conditions (see box 'What's in a word?' below). Names and labels are important because they are used as a sort of shorthand or jargon for what people understand about these conditions, so how other people talk about your condition, or your child's condition, will tell you a lot about where they are coming from in terms of what they understand. There has been a history of people also 'not wanting to label' children and young people, and while this was done with the best of intentions it can also be unhelpful if it delays getting the help that the child needs. The idea behind 'not labelling people' is that in developmental terms children and young people are still growing and changing physically and mentally, so giving them a medical label at an early age can stick with them for their whole lives and then be hard to change if this label, or diagnosis, is incorrect. This argument is fair for some conditions, particularly those that attract stigma, and probably is a guideline that should be used for some more clear mental health conditions. For example, the term 'Personality Disorder' is quite stigmatizing, and difficult to get rid of once it is in your medical history, and technically should not be used for people under 18, because personality is still developing. Some healthcare professionals will use 'Emerging Undiagnosed Personality Disorder' for children and young people, and this is also very unhelpful, especially as the latest thinking suggests that a lot of these problems can be better understood in terms of trauma experiences and people's ways of coping and surviving those experiences.

Neurodevelopmental conditions, however, are different from mental health problems that you develop later in life. You are born with a neurodevelopmental condition, and while it may change over your lifetime, and you learn to live with it, cope with the additional complications it gives to living your life, and may well to go on to thrive, it is actually part of you, and the 'neuro' bits of it are hard-wired in your brain. Understanding this helps the people around you to understand why some of the behaviours occur, because many of them are not easy to shift, and the way that neurodevelopmental conditions work may make it much harder for you to change your own behaviours. This is not to say that we can't work on them to help us cope with life better, but recognizing that having a neurodevelopment condition probably means you have a bit of an uphill struggle with changing things. This is where labels start to be helpful, because if you have a recognized label, or diagnosis, from a medical or healthcare professional, then people have to start to take the underlying difficulties seriously, and recognize that they need to do things differently to help you. In some administrations (including the UK) there are legal implications to having a diagnosis, which means that the education authorities have a legal duty to provide the additional help you need.

What a label can do is to give a pointer for what group of difficulties are most prominent, and what needs mostly to be taken into account. Currently the healthcare world likes to refer to everyone with autism as having 'Autism Spectrum Disorder' (ASD), although that covers a very wide range of people and older labels would use different labels that were a bit more specific. Asperger's Syndrome usually presents differently to people with Classic Autism for example. And none of these take into account what degree of learning disability a person has, either. For healthcare professionals, as well as social care staff and staff in education, these labels ought to give some idea of the type of difficulties – attentional problems with or without hyperactivity, for example – and a bit of a head start in thinking about how to help.

At the same time it is important to remember that everyone with any form of neurodevelopmental condition is different, and while they may have some symptomatic behaviour and thinking patterns that are common to other people with the same label, they are also individuals with different personalities and histories, which means they may react differently. This makes it a bit more difficult, especially for those in education (in my experience), to get their heads around the best ways to help.

What about 'neurodiversity'?

Having said that labels, or diagnoses, are important for helping to understand the group of symptoms that are likely, and that neurodevelopmental conditions are hardwired into the brain, there is an equally useful way of thinking about this which is generally called 'neurodiversity'. This was popularized in the book *Neurotribes* written by Steve Silberman (2015), mostly about autism, but generally working on the theory that humanity is actually made up of a very wide range of different sorts of people, so neurodevelopmental conditions ought to be seen as a normal part of that range, or spectrum, on which we all fit somewhere. This kind of thinking accepts difference in all its many forms, and fits in with how a lot of people think now about gender, for example. It also allows people to think in a more positive way about the positives that can come with neurodevelopmental difference; some people with autism are very focused, and this focus has led to scientific breakthroughs, some people with attentional problems are very creative and artistic, and finding a way to harness and use these strengths can be a better way of thinking.

There are many different terms that are used to describe autism; some of these are childhood autism, Asperger's and high functioning autism. Pervasive developmental disorder and pathological demand avoidance are used to describe difficulties that are considered part of the spectrum of autistic conditions. This range of conditions demonstrates the diversity across the autism spectrum. Similarly, there are a range of terms that describe attention difficulties; these include ADHD (Attention Deficit Hyperactivity Disorder), ADD (Attention Deficit Disorder and hyperkinetic disorder, and different neurodevelopmental conditions which include dyslexia, dyscalculia, Tourette's syndrome and dyspraxia which illustrate the wide range of conditions that are seen within the neurodevelopmental spectrum. These are only some of the conditions within the neurodiversity spectrum, which illustrates how wide and varied the conditions are. The important aspect to remember about all of these conditions is that they are hardwired into the brain and therefore, established as a condition for life. However, as children develop, the child's ability to manage their condition normally improves when moving in to adulthood.

How is anxiety different in neurodiverse people?

For neurodiverse people, there are two main issues that relate to anxiety that are important for to recognize: what is the source of the anxiety; and what is different about how to cope with it? The ideas, methods and techniques presented elsewhere in this book will all work for children and young people with neurodevelopmental conditions, but they may well be complicated by how the thinking process, in particular, is affected in each individual case.

What causes anxiety in neurodiverse children?

While the causes of anxiety in the neurodiverse child may be similar to those of other young people (trauma, bullying, worries about parents and friends, health anxieties or even climate change), the nature of the underlying condition may well play a much bigger part in understanding the reasons for anxiety than has previously been understood. There has been a common tendency to think, for example, that people with attentional problems just 'live in the moment' and aren't going to be worrying too much about what people think of them. This is a rather superficial way of understanding attentional problems; a better understanding would be to see that a cycle develops, which means that the impulsiveness or inattentiveness leads to a pattern of responses from other people that may contribute to anxiety. Particularly as young people with attentional problems grow older and more insightful to how people respond to their way of being, they notice these patterns, and can become anxious about the reactions that their behaviour gets from other people. For young people, who developmentally start to put more and more importance on their peer relationships, rather than family relationships, this often manifests itself in difficulty in making and maintaining effective relationships with their peers. The inattentiveness and inattention, which is part of the underlying condition, starts to be seen as immaturity by their natural friendship group, and often they will end up relating better to slightly younger children who can still relate to the spontaneity of this type of behaviour.

In the same way, the difficulty in maintaining good patterns of attention and performing as expected within the school environment can provoke anxiety. Difficulties in self-organization often become more evident, for example, on moving from a primary school environment to a secondary school where being able to follow a timetable (and not lose that timetable!), remember which building or classroom you are supposed to be in at any given time, and which day to bring in your sports gear etc., can lead to a pattern of negative interactions with staff, who often have a clear set of expectations for students dependent on their age. As this progresses, anxiety about relationships with peers, and with adults, can start to be tinged with anxiety about potential negative outcomes, and may lead to anxiety based issues such as reluctance to attend school in the form of school refusal or truanting (see Chapter 3).

For people on the autism spectrum the issues are likely to be related to not understanding what is expected of them, not being able to relate (again this becomes more important as young people grow older), or in being anxious about what comes next. The strong need for some people to stick to well understood routines is now better understood in this context, for example. If you are uncertain (because of your autism) about what is expected of you socially, in a new situation, or in a change of the normal routine, then this can be anxiety provoking. If you find the world to be a strange and threatening place, then changes to routine suddenly become very scary: how will you know what comes next and if it is safe? This level of stress and anxiety can become overwhelming and lead to the outburst (often called 'meltdowns') where the feelings that have built up inside become too much to cope with, leading to an almost primal expression of anguish which is very scary to the people around, as well as to the person who is experiencing it. Given that expressing emotions is difficult for people with autism it can take a long while to understand that some behaviours, like meltdowns, or avoidant behaviour (trying various strategies to get out of difficult situations) may well be caused by anxiety related to that underlying thinking process. For some people with autism and a lot of insight (and this applies more to girls than boys in general) the process of trying to act in an appropriate social manner in school, or elsewhere, can be very stressful and anxiety provoking, and the relief of coming home and being able to be yourself or live up to a different set of expectations, can also be very stressful. One young woman I knew – let's call her Alice – called this her 'fake self' at school, and her 'real self' at home, but she was extremely anxious during the time she was trying hard to be her 'fake self', and the longer she had to do this the harder it became for her to process why she had to do this, and to cope with the anxieties it caused in her. In extreme cases this anxiety can be literally crippling, causing people to be unable to move, or swallow, a condition known as catatonia, which is again thought to be caused largely by social anxiety.

Addressing the causes of anxiety

It makes sense then to try and first address the causes of the anxiety, and reduce the ones that make people anxious – prevention is better than cure, after all. Understanding the causes of stress and working around them will mean that actually having to deal with the stress is less frequent and leads to a calmer life.

This is easily said, but harder to put into practice. It may require both planning and adaptation for the young person and the family. Because routine and predictability may reduce stress and anxiety for people with various sorts of neurodiversity, planning ahead and preparing for situations, controlling the environment to which you or your child are exposed, will help. This isn't always completely possible, but knowing what the possible things are that are likely to reduce anxiety will help. Young people who are particularly sensitive to noise, for example, can wear ear defenders to dampen down the noise. Lots of supermarkets now have 'autism hours' where the background music is turned down or off, lighting is more subdued, and tannoy announcements are banned, for example, so if visiting the supermarket has always been anxiety provoking, and you have to take your child with you, then these measures can be very helpful. Likewise cinemas and theatres have increasingly been introducing special performances where the same adaptions are made; lower sound levels, less glaring lights etc. If you absolutely have to go to the fun fair (because everyone else is going) then daytime visits are less overwhelming than going when it is dark. Similarly days out are going to be easier if you have visited the attraction before, or if you do some research and familiarize yourself and have a plan before you go, so you and your child or young person have some idea of what to expect. Most museums and outdoor attractions (heritage railways, for example) have websites now with plans of the grounds, what is available, and what you can see and do. Prior planning of what you are going to encounter, which order you might like to do things while there, where the toilets are, and what you might be able to eat, will all reduce the anxiety likely to be provoked by going somewhere new.

For more routine daily life and school, then working around the worst stresses will start to become what is the new normal for you. It is hard to accept that you may not be able to do everything that other people take for granted. Ironically, spontaneity may not be the best thing for people with attentional problems, and certainly it is not for people with most forms of ASD, so the idea of planning ahead may be difficult, but if it reduces the anxieties and stresses, then it is better than the alternative, which may be traumatizing for everyone.

Adapting in other areas can be hard, especially if you have an ingrained idea that you have to treat all your children the same, a concept of fairness which is a bit skewed, because it doesn't take difference into account. While we can't remove all the stresses and anxiety provoking situations from life, we can certainly mitigate against many of them. School environments can be adapted to meet the particular needs of individuals, and each school, in the UK at least, will have a Special Educational Needs Coordinator (SENCO) to address this. Teachers sometimes fall into the trap of thinking they need to treat everyone the same, as they struggle with large classes, but actually educational theory does suggest that you should adapt to the needs of different pupils. Relatively simple issues like splitting activities into small sections, discreet reminders to return to task and frequent praise for small achievements will work very well with children with attentional difficulties, for example. Allowing the more restless to wander for a short period before returning to a task, will help them to refocus on the task and achieve the overall aim. For children and young people with sensory issues, arranging the environment of the classroom and facilities for breaks will all reduce the overall levels of stress and anxiety.

Using the ideas in this book with neurodiverse children

There will still be times when the anxiety becomes unbearable, so dealing with those times is also important. At the most extreme, the phenomenon known as 'meltdowns' represents the result of not being able to cope with this level of stress and anxiety. The National Autistic Society have done a very good video giving some insight into how this might be experienced (see the online support section at the end of the chapter), which is useful to watch. Meltdown behaviour can be difficult to cope with if you are a parent, relative or friend, but is even harder to experience yourself. Provided the individual is not harming themselves or others then it is probably best to let it run its course, and then be there for the person when they have exhausted themselves. Obviously if they are harming themselves or others you may need to intervene. The aim, therefore, should be to avoid getting to this extreme, so learning some techniques to reduce anxiety when it starts to build up, and break the cycle that leads to meltdown is important.

The techniques and ideas given elsewhere in this book will all still work, but they may be harder to apply. For people with attentional problems, and particularly those with poor impulse control, the process of the anxiety building and becoming too difficult to cope with may be very quick, and levels of insight into this starting to happen may be very low too, depending on age and maturity. Younger children in particular, have very little control over their emotional responses, and while this changes, as a normal developmental process for everyone as we learn to adapt and understand our feelings, it can take much longer for people with attentional difficulties. This process may need to be taught, or the young person helped to be more aware of trigger situations, or understanding how their own body reacts or changes as they start to feel more anxious. Teaching this, or helping young people to develop self-awareness of their own bodies and their emotional responses is part of many techniques, but again the attentional issues may make it much harder; effectively they may have less time in which to stop and think what is happening to them because of their inbuilt impulsiveness. This is not to say that it isn't possible, just that the process of learning and being able to use the normal tools may be considerably harder, and take longer than for other children and young people. And again this is not their 'fault', it's just the way they are.

For people on the autism spectrum the issues may be different, especially if they have what is called 'concrete thinking', a lack of flexibility around concepts and abstract thinking. Your child might have very strong ideas, for example, about what is 'fair' and 'not fair', and may find it hard to see things from other perspectives. Likewise, a lot of Cognitive Behavioural Therapy techniques rely on changing how we think about something, particularly something we are anxious about, and then changing the behaviour around that concept and the behaviour associated with it. If you have the kind of mind that has a fairly fixed idea about things, then this process may well take a lot longer, or be extremely difficult to achieve. Alice, whom we met earlier, had a lot of issues, when I saw her over a very long period, with coming to terms with the idea that her autism made her 'different' to others, rather than in her mind 'bad' because she wasn't normal (by her standards). Helping her to think of herself as 'different' but that this was okay, as a way of coping with her own thoughts, took a very long time because of the fixed nature of her thinking. In Alice's case getting a formal diagnosis was part of this process, but it was a very bumpy road. This is very individual to each young person, so for staff working with young people it is important that they take the time to get to know each young person as an individual, and tailor their approaches to the individual needs of that person.

Self-stimulating behaviours

'Stimming' is the usual description of self-stimulating behaviours, and these can often increase when a child or young person is anxious. They can, and often do, also occur as an expression of happiness, so it can be confusing to the outside observer. For people with autism the most common stims are hand-flapping, moving fingers in front of the eyes, clapping or making repetitive sounds. If this happens unexpectedly it can take others aback and lead to stigmatizing looks and other negative expressions from the uninformed. There are some forms of stimming which are self-harmful, such as head-banging or slapping or punching yourself – these should be seen as a symptom of distress, and addressed as such. For most stimming behaviours, however, it is better to see this as a coping mechanism, and if it is not harming anyone else then it is best to accept and understand it as just that. If the stimming is suppressed (by someone repeatedly telling your child not to do it, for example), then it is likely that an alternative coping mechanism will develop. In therapeutic terms removing one coping mechanism (however undesirable) without helping to develop different ways of coping is almost always disastrous – the new method may be worse.

Other 'disabilities'

We've mostly looked so far at people living with ADHD and autism. For other neurodevelopmental conditions the causes of anxiety are going to be either about other people's reactions to your child as a person who presents as 'different', or your child's own adjustment to their identity as a person who is shaped in part by this difference. People with tic disorders such as Tourette's often find that their tics are more prominent when they are anxious or stressed, but if this leads to an increase in the tics, or they are the kind of verbal tics that are socially inappropriate then the circular pattern begins again: the more you try to stop the tics, the worse they become. For people with physically obvious differences, the reactions that are routinely encountered can lead to anxiety or avoidant behaviours. If your experience of being in a wheelchair has been that many people are patronising to you, or that simple activities of daily life, like accessing buildings, finding an appropriate toilet and so on, are all difficult, then one reaction would be to start to avoid the activities that make you anxious.

For young people who develop illnesses, rather than being born with something that makes them 'different', this can also be anxiety provoking. The 'adjustment reaction' of getting a diabetes diagnosis as a teenager, for example, can be a very difficult time in coming to terms with this new aspect of your identity that has been suddenly thrust upon you. Particularly in the teenage years, when – ironically – finding out who you are as an individual carries with it an element of need to conform to a peer-pressured concept of normality, this can lead to high degrees of anxiety and even some self-destructive behaviour (which we will talk about in more in Chapter 14). This sudden change in understanding that you have a life-long condition that you have to learn to live with, rather than what you had hoped and dreamed of, can be very difficult to cope with in a time when feelings are extreme and strongly felt. Growing up is about learning to cope with some of these feelings, and finding ways to self-regulate and get through life, so for many young people this is the first time they will have had to cope with such an earth-shattering experience.

What else helps?

Alongside the need for routines and predictability, the need for consistency is really important. If a child or young person is met with one approach at home, and a different way of doing things at school, then confusion about expectations leads to increased anxiety. This also applies to extended families, stepfamilies, grandparent attitudes, weekends with non-custodial parents, and a host of other settings that are likely to be encountered. Developing a consistent approach across these different settings is important for all children, but while children without these challenges may be able to work out that the rules are different when they stay with dad or mum and their new partner are different from the usual rules at their main family home, this is much harder for this group. Likewise there may be differences of opinion between generations, and while the parents have to learn to adapt to the particular needs of their children it can be harder for grandparents, who see them less, to fully understand why they need to react to this child differently to their other grandchildren. Children and young people spend a significant part of their lives at school, so getting consistency of method and approach between the two settings is also important to lower levels of anxiety. As a personal example of this, my own two boys (who both have learning difficulties and ASD) went to a school that taught them to use Makaton sign language to communicate. They didn't teach Makaton to us, so the boys started to get very frustrated when they started signing, and we couldn't understand what they were trying to tell us!

Remember, everyone living with neurodiversity is different, and some of these ideas may be helpful, but what works best for each young person will vary according to their own individual needs. Hopefully some of these ideas will be useful in helping to understand what those individual needs are, and how they can be helped.

References and further reading

Baldwin, L. (ed.) (2020) *Nursing Skills for Children and Young People's Mental Health*. Switzerland: Springer.

Silberman, S. (2015) *Neurotribes: The Legacy of Autism and How to Think Smarter About People who Think Differently*. New York: Allen & Unwin.

Online resources

British Dyslexia Association: <www.bdadyslexia.org.uk> Also has a good video on neurodiversity: <www.bdadyslexia.org.uk/dyslexia/neurodiversity-and-co-occurring-differences/what-is-neurodiversity>

Mind Ed (educational resource): <www.minded.org.uk>

National Attention Deficit Information and Support Service: <www.addiss.co.uk>

National Autistic Society: <www.autism.org.uk> Also NAS video on sensory overload: <www.youtube.com/watch?v=aPknwW8mPAM>

Tourettes Action: <www.tourettes-action.org.uk>

Young Minds: <www.youngminds.org.uk>

6

Anxieties about eating

Delysia McKnight, Social Worker & CBT Therapist

This chapter looks at what difficulties with eating means, what sort of eating difficulties your child might experience and what you can do to help them.

When you first notice your child is not eating it can, of course, be very worrying (feeding your child is often seen as a primary function of being a parent), but in most instances it is just a phase, and with consistent guidance and boundaries it will pass. However, sometimes it will be something more, and your child will need a bit more support.

You will have heard the terms 'eating difficulties' and 'eating disorder'; what differentiates the two is *impact*. Young people and adults can often develop a problem with eating, anxiety or mood, and this resolves itself without the need for any professional input, and does not greatly impact on their life or well-being. It was a problem, and stopped being a problem. However, if what your child is doing is having a significant impact on their life, be that physical, psychological or social, then it can be viewed as a disorder – it is causing *disorder* in that person's life. The terms are often used interchangeably, which can lead to some confusion.

It can be difficult to diagnose an eating disorder in children and adolescents. This is partly due to the number of eating problems that can occur in very early childhood with feeding and weaning. (Bryant-Waugh, 2020). Fussy eating is commonplace in pre-school children and may even result in some weight loss, but it often resolves itself and can indeed be looked at as a phase of development. Introducing new foods, textures and tastes to children as they develop is a usual way to increase food variety. This is a natural phenomena when children move from milk to solids in their early years; trying different foods to see which they like and dislike. Continuing this through life is helpful to keep children's food variety increasing and there is less likelihood for fussy eating. However, as a child develops, persistent eating difficulties are not commonplace and there may be something more going on. This may not be an eating disorder as such, but other issues that your child is dealing with that could be impacting upon their appetite and their eating.

It is important to rule out any physical issues that could affect eating. Constipation, acid reflux, food intolerances and toothache can all make eating difficult and indeed cause some anxiety around food. Speaking to your GP in the first instance is really important. At the appointment, it can be useful to have a list of concerns and what you have noticed to ensure it's a productive consultation. Additionally, if you think this might be more than a phase, again, keeping a note of symptoms and behaviours is useful (we will look at signs and symptoms later in the chapter). If you are anything like me, when I speak to my GP I always forget half of what I planned to tell them!

Before we look at the different types of eating difficulties/disorders, it's important to have an understanding of what is a normal, healthy weight. There is no simple answer to that one! Guidelines suggest that with children and young people we look at the height, age weight and sex of the child to tell us where they are sitting based on the average. This is the information you find in the 'red book' (given to all parents after their baby's birth), and it is often used to determine where a young person is in relation to the general population and to build a picture of their development. In essence what a weight and height chart shows is where a child sits compared to the rest of the population of the same age. For example, if your child is right in the middle, so that 50 per cent of children that age are taller and 50 per cent are shorter, they are said to be on the 50th percentile. It is not foolproof, and health is about more than a number on a scale or a percentage on a chart, but it can gives us something to work with and see how a child is developing.

For people aged 18 and above we use BMI (Body Mass Index) to determine a healthy weight for height. While there is some discussion around where the bottom of this should be, on the whole the below is recognized:

- Underweight: below 18.5.
- Healthy weight: 18.5–24.9.

- Overweight: 25.0–29.9.
- Obese: over 30.0.

There is some debate about the lower end of the range of normal as most people do not sit naturally at a BMI 18.5 and there is often some restriction and restraint needed to maintain this BMI – however, there are always exceptions to this rule. The same applies to the upper end of healthy weight – some people will sit naturally above 25, and that is healthy for them. 'Set point' is what we refer to when we think about where a person's body weight sits easily without too much being needed in terms of controlling intake and activity – this is different for everybody and some may sit outside the recognized ranges. As a reference point, it is of course only relevant once all development has stopped and the person has reached a stable adult weight. In addition, people from ethnic populations (e.g. Asian young people) often sit naturally at a lower BMI and therefore may fall in the underweight category, but this is not unhealthy for them. BMI is a useful tool, but it has its limitations. It is also important to note where a person's weight has been, where it has fallen to, and what the rate of loss has been in assessing the risks associated with weight loss. For example, a person may have lost a considerable amount of weight but remain in the healthy weight band – it may be assumed that this is fine, but in fact the body may struggle with the physical impact of fast weight loss.

Types of eating problems/difficulties

Anorexia Nervosa (AN)

Obsessive desire to lose weight by refusing to eat/limiting food intake and over-exercising. Over evaluation of weight and shape in relation to how the person sees/judges themselves.

Bulimia Nervosa (BN)

Obsessive desire to lose weight by extreme bouts of fasting/restricting followed by episodes of binging and then self-induced vomiting.

Other Specified Feeding or Eating Disorder (OSFED)/Eating Disorder Not Otherwise Specified (EDNOS)

Anorexia Nervosa and Bulimia Nervosa are diagnosed when someone meets the criteria of behavioural, psychological and physical symptoms. However, sometimes a person does not meet all of the criteria and when this happens they might be diagnosed with an 'Other Specified Feeding or Eating Disorder' (OSFED). This was previously known as 'Eating Disorder Not Otherwise Specified' (EDNOS). Sometimes also referred to as atypical AN or BN.

The impact of OSFED is every bit as serious as anorexia and bulimia, and requires treatment. OSFED accounts for a large percentage of all eating disorders diagnosed. An example of OSFED would be atypical anorexia where someone may have the thoughts, feelings and behaviours associated with anorexia but their weight is in a normal range. In atypical bulimia it could be that the person has all the symptoms of bulimia but the occurrence of binging and purging is not as frequent.

Pica

This is classified as a mental disorder where people eat non-food items such as dirt, cloth or chalk. It's not the same as when a person will eat non-food items in order to trick the hunger signals.

Rumination Disorder

This is a mental disorder where the person will regurgitate food and either re-chew, re-swallow or spit it out. Often this develops as a way to manage emotions. This is different from chewing food and then spitting it out, which is usually an attempt to have the taste of food but avoid the calories.

Orthorexia

This is a descriptive term and is not a formally recognized disorder, but understanding of the condition is being developed through research. It is characterized by an obsession with healthy eating, to the cost of other food groups that are viewed as unhealthy, often to the point that the person is underweight and/or suffering from malnutrition.

Avoidant Restrictive Food Intake Disorder (ARFID)

This a formal diagnosis and is where a person fails to eat or accept an adequate diet in terms of energy and/or nutrient intake and as a result there is significant impairment to health, development and/or general functioning. Restriction is not related to weigh/shape as with Anorexia or Bulimia Nervosa but rather more to do with a lack of interest, or sensory aspects of food, texture, appearance, for example (Bryant-Waugh, 2020).

The impact of eating disorders

Eating disorders are functional – they serve a purpose and often they serve multiple purposes. Below are some of the reasons young people have told us about how their eating disorder is helping them:

I feel like I need to punish myself.
It helps me to achieve a sense of control and safety.
I want to avoid being judged badly by others.
It gives me a sense of achievement and feeling successful.
It means I don't have to worry about other things as it takes all my focus.

With anorexia nervosa, bulimia nervosa and FEDOS, it is important to remember that they have more in common than that which separates them. All stem from a deep unhappiness with weight, shape and appearance. Any child with any of these disorders will judge themselves on how well they think they are doing at changing these features and will feel judged by others in relation to this. Low weight can result in an increased physical risk, but so can frequent purging, and anyone with these conditions will experience a negative impact on their psychological and social well-being.

The Minnesota Project, carried out in the 1940s, illustrates the impact of starvation on a person.

The Minnesota Project

The Minnesota study (Keys et al., 1950) on the effects of semi-starvation showed what happened when 36 men's calorie intake was restricted to a point where their weight dropped to 75 per cent of their pre-starvation weight. It is important to note that these men were all tested to ensure they were healthy from a physical, psychological and social perspective. The men were observed prior to the restriction – many were outgoing, had girlfriends, hobbies, and so on. As their weight dropped, what was observed was a loss of interest in activities, relationships ending – they also became more irritable. Their focus turned to food and eating, some made strange concoctions, played with their food, some even began to hoard food in their rooms.

These behaviours are often what we see in children or young people who are restricting their intake or attempting to under-eat consistently. This is why, in the first instance, it is so important to begin with re-establishing a regular intake of food and regaining a healthy weight (if applicable). By doing so we can reduce the child's symptoms, to begin to look at what may have triggered the eating difficulties in the first place, and find alternative, helpful ways to manage them better.

Psychological impact

As undereating and/or being underweight persists, difficulty with concentration and focus is noted; making decisions becomes more difficult as the mind is preoccupied with thoughts of food and appearance. Mood tends to lower and, as noted above, most people become more irritable. Rigidity can be seen either in thinking or in behaviours and routine, and change is more difficult to tolerate.

Social impact

As your child becomes more focused on food, eating and weight there is less 'space' for other things such as their hobbies, interests and friendships. They might become more withdrawn as they don't have the energy or interest to maintain relationships and, as social interactions often revolve around food or going to places that have food, such social occasions may become too hard for them, leading to avoidance. This of course will have further negative impact on their mood, and so the circle continues.

What can cause eating difficulties/disorders?

Psychological factors

Some of these might include low self-esteem, perfectionism, feeling inadequate, lacking control in life, low mood, anxiety or trauma.

Social factors

Social factors may come from cultural/societal pressures to 'look good' and 'fit in' with norms, or from involvement in a sport/activity that emphasizes body image.

Interpersonal factors

Such factors would include difficulties in relationships with others (conflict/abuse/bullying), and difficulties expressing or managing emotions.

As you can see, there are very many reasons behind the development of difficulties with food and weight. You might find it useful to look at eating disorders as a coping mechanism when someone is feeling overwhelmed by either difficult emotions or situations. Eating difficulties do not emerge out of the blue and they do have a purpose – your child is not just being difficult, or awkward. A good starting point is to try and find out if things have changed at school, with friends, or whether there is something they are worrying about – and to help them find solutions for this. You have a wealth of experience and knowledge that can help and perhaps stop the eating difficulties becoming something more. However, sometimes more help is needed – and we will be looking at some strategies that you might find useful here.

What separates an eating disorder from other disorders is the focus on weight, shape and food, and also on the following: first, how your child judges themselves according to how well they are controlling this; second, a refusal to be at a normal weight for their age/height; and third, a fear of gaining weight. Other disorders such as low mood and anxiety can affect eating patterns and routines, but the drive here is different.

There are, of course, more complex factors involved as well – such as the role of biology, of chemicals in the brain, and of brain development. CAT scans (scans that show the inside of the body) have shown us that the brain of someone with anorexia nervosa lights up differently when shown pictures of food; additionally, chemical imbalances have been found in levels of serotonin and dopamine, and the chemicals have an impact on both mood and appetite. In people with diagnosed eating disorders, levels of these are lower than normal. This chapter does not have the scope to delve into these findings, but there are some further reading recommendations at the end of the chapter if you want to learn more about it.

What to look out for

There are numerous lists of signs and symptoms available on the internet, and no single one is exhaustive, but there are some things that the research tells us can be indicators that difficulties with food, weight and/or appearance may be developing. The main ones include:

Changes in mood, withdrawing from family and friends.
Being more irritable, especially around meal times.
Saying they have eaten already.
Disappearing to the bathroom after meals.
Exercising more than normal.
Starting to drop food groups, such as carbohydrates, pasta, potatoes and sweet foods. (Not all will do this – some will eat a wide range of foods but will eat smaller amounts than before.)
Saying they are not hungry more than normal (appetite can change – and that is normal – but it becomes concerning if it is persistent, or if your child seems to be avoiding eating).
Being more self-critical, making negative statements about themselves.
Avoiding eating with others.
More interest in what is in their meals, and in the calories and/or fat content.

Consequences of eating difficulties/disorders that go unchecked

It is important to address eating difficulties/disorders as they can have very real consequences both physically and emotionally if left unchecked. Persistent low weight can impact upon growth, bone health, menstrual cycle or onset of puberty. Chronic low weight can lead to damage to internal organs, muscle loss and osteoporosis.

Self-induced vomiting associated with bulimia nervosa can damage teeth, throat, stomach and again – if it happens over a number of years – stress can be placed on the heart as vomiting upsets the levels of potassium in our body. Potassium creates the electrical current that sparks the heart.

While all of this does sound frightening, it is reversible with the establishment of regular eating, normal weight and stopping the binge/purge cycle of bulimia.

Myths

Eating disorders are not ...
  ... your fault.
  ... your child being stubborn.
  ... your child trying to punish you or be difficult.
  ... a dislike of food itself – most people with eating disorders love food, but it has become tangled up in their fear and worries.
  ... attention-seeking.
  ... a case of 'if they just ate, they would be fine'.
  Another myth is that you must do whatever you can not to upset or annoy your child – this is an important one – in order to help your child you will need to upset and annoy them.

Strategies for dealing with eating difficulties/disorders

So, it seems that this is more than a passing phase. What do you do now? How do you approach this? It will depend on the age of your child – if your child is younger, you will need to be directive, and set boundaries around eating, while not turning every meal into a battlefield – this is easier said than done.

With an older child, broach the subject gently but firmly. Using statements such as 'I've noticed' (refer back to earlier advice about keeping a log of behaviours you have noticed) or 'I'm worried that …'. They may not accept this, and often those with eating problems do not believe there is one, so again a gentle but firm approach is needed. Do not ignore it just because you do not want to upset or cause arguments.

Keep talking. Once there is more acceptance – or at least not so much resistance – then it becomes a case of working together to begin to resolve the issue.

Food is the prescription and the medicine

Dealing with eating difficulties can create a lot of frustration, upset and stress. Throughout this, it is important to always blame the illness for the difficulties, not yourself, or your child. It will be difficult for your child to make decisions and choices so plan ahead for what you are going to have at each meal, and agree meal times in the first instance. Later on, you can work on being flexible but at the beginning, the most important thing is to get a regular eating pattern established again.

Managing meal times

- Meal times are often the most difficult for all involved, so it is better to plan ahead. There can be some options allowed, but keep these to a minimum, as too many options will cause anxiety for your child. As well as planning meals, plan the shopping list and agree who is doing what.
- Be clear about what is expected, and stick to a timeframe for each meal. Thirty to 40 minutes for main meals, and 15 minutes for snacks is usually recommended.
- Prompt your child when needed, for example, if they haven't started eating or they're putting their fork down – you can validate them by saying things like, 'I know how difficult this is, but you need to start now.'
- Keep the conversation light, using it as a good distraction and avoiding food related topics.

- Be patient – this difficulty did not develop overnight, and it won't resolve overnight. Your child will respond best to a gentle but firm approach – this is what feels safe for most children and young people.
- Be consistent and do not get into debates or negotiations, this distracts from the task – which is to eat.
- Some families find it is better to eat together, but for others the child might need a space on their own to start with, transitioning to eat with family once they have established a better eating routine.
- Be observant – it is very easy for food to be thrown in the bin, put up sleeves or given to the dog. I know it can be very difficult to imagine that your child might act in this way around food, but remember it's the illness driving this behaviour, not your child.
- Be aware of behaviours that can hinder eating such as using small plates or utensils, pushing food around the plate, or mixing it together to make it look as if more has been eaten.
- After the meal it is important to distract your child with activities, to help them not think too much about what they have eaten. It is better if this is an activity that can be done sitting down – something that involves using hands and is mentally absorbing, like crafts and puzzles.
- If you suspect that your child is purging after eating, it is important that you prevent them from going to the bathroom either during or straight after meals for at least 30–45 minutes. By this time the urge to purge has often declined and it also allows time for the body to start digesting the food (making it ineffective as a means of weight control) and get the nutrition it needs, reducing the damage to the stomach, throat and teeth.
- It can be helpful to keep diaries or accounts, we professionals love them! You know your child better than we do, you see them every day, whereas if your child is receiving help at an outpatient clinic, chances are this is once a week. Your records can provide really useful information and insight into daily routines, when things are most difficult, what is working and what is not.

Think about your own support, about who is around you that you can talk to, moan to or vent – all of this is normal, and valid (see Chapter 2 for strategies on looking after yourself). As we have seen, when you talk to your child it is always better to refer to the illness using whatever language works best for you, rather than to their behaviour (in therapy you may even be asked to give the illness a name, in order to help create a separation between illness and child).

It is completely understandable to get angry or frustrated with your child, but aiming your anger at them and not their illness could lead to your child hiding more, allow disordered eating to develop more, and for thoughts and behaviours to become more embedded.

Change will and should be small at this point. If you are not receiving professional help at this time then any changes to your child's food intake should be small. If your child has not eaten anything at all for a few days (more than two days), you should seek medical advice.

Little and often is usually best

Work together with your partner, if you have one. This way, there is less room for slip-ups and, as with all parenting, it is better to give a united front. This creates safety and boundaries, which are important. We know that every family is different and works in different ways, so the information and guidance in this chapter is designed in such a way that you can take from it and find what works for you and your child.

It is important to be available at meal times to support and encourage. This may mean a change in your or your partner's working pattern; or you can ask a significant other to help with this. Grandparents can often provide great support, if appropriate.

Involving the school and letting them know your concerns can also be helpful as most schools have a pastoral department that can become involved with, and help with, observations, support lunch times, and provide a quiet room to have lunch in.

Eva Musby (2014) has a great book which has loads of strategies, tips and advice based on her own experience with her daughter and she also has videos available online. Details are at end of the chapter.

Being proactive – creating a good body image

Here are some of the things that we know about body image and what can impact negatively on it. According to the Dove Self Esteem Project:

- The world of fashion – 60 minutes looking at a magazine lowers the self-esteem of 80 per cent of young people and women.
- Current media ideals of thinness are naturally achievable by less than 5 per cent of the female population. We are setting ourselves up for failure.
- Young people are bombarded by images of the 'perfect' body, life, product.
- On average a young person sees between 400–600 adverts per day.

Social media/online influence

There are a growing number of sites online often referred to as 'pro-ana' or 'pro-mia' which stands for 'pro' anorexia and 'pro' bulimia. The term 'thinspiration' is also widely used in the media. These sites promote anorexia and bulimia nervosa as lifestyle choices. They usually have an online community, tips and advice on how to achieve a weight loss goal. Online stories where people are blogging their daily intake can be positive, but the young people we work with tell us that sometimes when you look at the comments left, they are very negative about what the person is eating, or the amount of food consumed. Like all social media it has two sides. Talk to your child about the dangers of online sites and how to keep safe online. If you are concerned that your child is following unhelpful social media or online communities, talk to them about the dangers and remind them how to stay safe. Organizations such as the NSPCC and Barnardo's have a number of great resources you can use to have a discussion with your child. Boundaries might have to be set about time spent online and where on the internet they are. It is difficult, as there are so many ways to access sites, (phone, tablets and televisions) but it is worth the battle to make sure your child is not online late at night or unsupervised and accessing sites that might be promoting unsafe eating behaviours. Internet matters (<www.internetmatters.org/>) is also a really helpful site to support parents managing their children's online activities. It is also important to remind your child that the images they are scrolling through on their phones are, more often than not, altered and not a true reflection of the person featured – rather, they are pushing an unrealistic version of life, a perfect weight, shape or lifestyle.

It should also be said, of course, that we are not entirely sure of the impact of social media on the development of eating difficulties. As we have seen, there are many factors that contribute to their development. While social media can contribute to how unhappy children feel about their appearance, it is important to consider other factors contributing to their difficulties, such as school, friendships or home lives. As more research is conducted we will continue to get a better understanding of the impact of social media, both positive and negative.

Boys and negative body image

When we think about body image, we immediately think about the pressure on girls, however, this also affects boys too. The advertising think tank Credos' report 'A picture of health' surveyed 1005 boys between 8 and 18 years of age and found that many of them felt they needed to look better and they felt a pressure to do something about it, as much as their female peers. Some boys were not aware that the media enhanced pictures of males as much as females. There is a similar lack of awareness in identifying body image and eating difficulties in boys. It is important not to overlook these difficulties in boys.

So, how do we stop the tide?

Fostering a positive body image

- Try to demonstrate a healthy approach to eating behaviours. This is really about balance – it is not saying that losing weight is wrong, but that it is only needed if your weight is having a negative impact on your health not appearance.

- Step away from the idea of bad foods. There is no such thing; it is more about moderate amounts and having a balanced diet. When you deny yourself a food because you see it is as bad or unhealthy, that will be the one you think about the most! Not labelling food in this way helps ensure a positive relationship with food. The message is about how to nourish your body and mind.
- Focus on non-appearance related traits. In an office, once one person says a negative thing about themselves everyone else joins in about themselves – and the impact? Within five minutes we are all feeling rubbish! Praise and encourage other traits, behaviours, successes.
- Talk about the impact of media pictures, and fashion. The Dove campaign for real beauty is a great site that you can look at with your child, and has loads of information and advice on how the beauty/fashion industry works, and how to help your child develop a positive body image (details for the website are at the end of this chapter).
- Highlight aspects of people that are attractive apart from their weight and looks – note whether they are confident, funny or organized, for example.
- It's a tough time for young people; you can help them see that bodies come in all shapes and sizes.
- If your child is overweight, help them get more active rather than focus on calories, and help them make better choices or balance it out at home.

It's a difficult area and you will get it wrong sometimes – that's normal!

Look after yourself!

Finally, a few words on looking after yourself. This can be a very daunting and challenging time for all the family, so it is important that wherever possible time is taken to maintain normality, and to do activities that are not associated with meal times. Take time out for yourself, use your support network, family and friends to support you wherever possible.

References and further reading

Bryant-Waugh, R. (2020) *ARFID Avoidant Restrictive Food Intake Disorder: A Guide for Parents and Carers*. London: Routledge.

Dove Self Esteem Project. Women in the media: give the stereotypes a makeover. <www.dove.com/uk/dove-self-esteem-project/help-for-parents/media-and-celebrities/women-in-the-media.html>

Fairburn, C.G. (2008) *Cognitive Behavior Therapy and Eating Disorders*. New York: Guildford Press.

Keys, A., Brazek, J., Henschel, A., Mickelsen, O. and Taylor, H.L. (1950) *The Biology of Human Starvation* (two volumes). Minneapolis: University of Minnesota Press.

Locke, J. and Le Grange, D. (2005) *Help Your Teenager Beat an Eating Disorder*. New York: Guildford Press.

Musby, E. (2014) *Anorexia and Other Eating Disorders. How to Help Your Child Eat Well and Be Well*. APRICA.

Schmidt, U., Startup, H. and Treasure, J. (2019) *A Cognitive Interpersonal Therapy Workbook for Treating Anorexia Nervosa: The Maudsley Model*. London: Routledge.

Seubert A. and Virdi, P. (2019) *Trauma Informed Approaches to Eating Disorders*. New York: Springer.

Treasure, J., Smith, G. and Crane, A. (2017) *Skills-based Caring for a Loved One with an Eating Disorder. The New Maudsley Method* (Second Edition). London: Routledge.

Online resources

Eva Musby – Helping you free your child of an eating disorder: <anorexia-family.com>. Website run by Eva Musby, based on her own experiences, offering advice and guidance.

Bodywhys: <www.bodywhys.ie> National Irish charity for eating disorders.

Beat: <www.b-eat.co.uk> National UK charity for eating disorders.

FEAST: <www.feast-ed.org> Website providing good advice and guidance on eating disorders.

Dove: <dove.com> Another good website for factsheets, activities to help build self-esteem and body confidence.

Maudsley Parents: <www.maudsleyparents.org>. A site for parents offering information on eating disorders and the family based treatment approach.

7

Social anxiety: worries about being judged by others

Ben Lea, RMN & CBT Therapist

This chapter explores anxieties associated with being judged by others, which we will refer to as social anxiety or social phobia. We will explore what social anxieties are, who it impacts, signs you should look out for, and what you can do to help your child. Experiencing worries about being judged by others is a normal part of adolescent development, when young people are finding their place in the world and social pressures are increasing around them. Social media now plays a significant part of modern life, where the impression is that other people have a perfect life, never make mistakes, and look great all of the time. As a result, most children, teenagers and young people find it difficult to live up to these expectations or perceptions.

While experiencing social anxieties is a normal aspect of development in adolescence, it can also develop into quite a significant and debilitating problem and even into a social phobia. Social phobia is described as 'a marked and persistent fear of social performance in which embarrassment may occur' (American Psychiatric Association, 2013). This can impact people in different ways, but there will often be an immediate and significant fear of exposure to social situations. The child may seek to avoid social situations or endure them with dread. Although they may well still attend school or family functions, they will do so reluctantly. Prior to these social situations, they may experience very high levels of anxiety and stress, sometimes leading to panic attacks prior to or at the event.

Signs of social anxiety before or during these situations can manifest themselves through concerns around being judged by others, or worries about their performance. They may lead to worries or fears about people seeing physical signs that they are anxious, such as going incredibly red or blushing, shaking profusely or a trembling voice.

Children with social anxiety difficulties may also attempt to dissect and evaluate their social performance following a social encounter. Their heightened state of anxiety and their focus on the negative aspects of the social encounter may well drive a further spiralling of anxiety levels, which leads to difficulties in their emotional state.

Is social anxiety impacting my child?

The easiest way to determine if this is something which is part of normal development or an indication of a moderate to significant problem is to think about how it affects the child's life:

- Does it stop them from doing the things they should or would like to be doing?
- Do they struggle with going to school due to these anxieties?
- Are they not making friends, or are they keeping friends at arm's length?
- Do they avoid parties or extended family members, and does this affect other aspects of their mental health such as their mood – a common problem if someone is experiencing difficulties with a form of social anxiety?

The prevalence of social anxiety increases quite drastically in the pre-adolescent and early adolescent years, resulting in an increase in the onset of social phobia, which peaks at approximately aged 15.

A study found the rate of social anxiety was less than half a per cent in 12–13-year-olds, and rose to 2 per cent in 14–15-year-olds. Studies have also found that these rates of social anxiety increased across the 14–17-year-old age group to 4 percent and more than doubled for 18–24-year-olds to over 8 per cent (NHS Digital, 2017).

I'm sure most parents can remember their own childhood experiences during their pre-teen and adolescent years. It's a very difficult time in development: there are pressures from school and from parents, and social pressures are also very high at a time when peer groups might be less understanding and caring to one another. In fact, research suggests that at least a quarter of children report extreme forms of bullying from peers.

There is no one factor which would identify who is more at risk of developing problems with social anxiety, however we are aware that people who might have had reduced opportunities to develop relationships with others, but also experienced peer victimization, are more at risk of developing social anxieties. Examples of this could include a young person who lives in a very rural area and has had limited opportunities for social interaction with others outside of their family, or a child who has been subjected to ongoing bullying with their school. Social interactions require quite complex skills, and if children have had limited or negative experiences with peers, they may then focus on the threat or fears that arise in these social interactions, such as signs of disapproval from others as a result of past experiences or a perceived lack of opportunities.

There are also the physical signs associated with anxiety which can include a racing heart, increased respiratory rate, shaking, sweating and an upset stomach. These things can feel overwhelming, and might result in a child focusing on these symptoms, instead of paying attention to the social interaction itself and developing their skills.

When this happens, children are understandably going to want to avoid these experiences or use behaviours (safety behaviours) which make them stand out less or make them feel more comfortable. We also know that these safety behaviours – such as not making eye contact, keeping their head down, not talking and so on – can contaminate social interactions and uninventively draw more attention to themselves, making them less likeable to their peers.

We also know that avoiding anxiety is not helpful in the long term and that, because of their avoidance, children with social anxiety are less likely to have friends or to involve themselves in exactly the type of extracurricular activities that would help them learn that social interactions and relationships are not as scary as they perceive them to be.

Signs parents can look out for

A child with social anxiety difficulties may struggle with particular thoughts prior, during and following social interactions with others. These thoughts might include:

Before a social interaction: 'What if I make a mistake? I might not have anything to say, I might trip up, and I'll go bright red.'
During a social interaction: 'Everyone is staring at me, I'm shaking, this is going terribly, no one likes me.'
Following a social interaction: 'I made a fool of myself, they must have been laughing at me when I left, I wish I had never gone.'

The thoughts that they might experience during social interactions will induce behaviours and signs that you as a parent can look out for, if you're wondering if your child is struggling with social anxiety.

Every child is different, and it is helpful to keep an open mind when you think about the list of signs below – there could in fact be other difficulties that your child is experiencing which may result in some of these behaviours. Examples of these difficulties include academic problems, low mood or bullying, all of which could result in your child not wanting to participate in particular activities.

Key signs of social anxiety in a child

- Avoidance of peer groups and social activities.
- Avoidance of school.
- Avoidance of family gatherings.
- Difficulties in attending shops and an avoidance of paying for items.
- Avoidance of public transport.
- Wanting parent to be present when leaving the home.
- Presenting with physical signs of anxiety prior, during and following social situations.
- Having few or no friends.
- Fear of being late, due to the increased attention drawn to self.
- Low mood.
- Difficulties with sleep.

- Possible improvements in mood during weekends and school holidays, when social interactions are reduced and the child's anxieties decrease.

Although these are the main signs to look out for, there are also diagnostic guidelines created by the American Psychiatric Association which clinicians use to determine if someone meets the criteria for a social anxiety disorder (*Diagnostic and Statistical Manual of Mental Disorders: DSM-V*). It can sometimes be useful to think about these diagnostic symptoms when talking to your GP or local children's mental health service to help with supporting and providing evidence if you want a referral for your child for further support.

These guidelines can also be useful to share with your child, as this can help them make sense of their own experiences and to understand that their difficulties are recognized by others.

American Psychiatric Association definition of social phobia

A. A persistent fear of one or more social or performance situations in which the person is exposed to unfamiliar people or to possible scrutiny by others. The individual fears that he or she will act in a way (or show anxiety symptoms) that will be embarrassing and humiliating.

B. Exposure to the feared situation almost invariably provokes anxiety, which may take the form of a situationally bound or situationally pre-disposed panic attack.

C. The person recognizes that this fear is unreasonable or excessive.

D. The feared situations are avoided, or else are endured with intense anxiety and distress.

E. The avoidance, anxious anticipation, or distress in the feared social or performance situation(s) interferes significantly with the person's normal routine, occupational (academic) functioning, or social activities or relationships, or there is marked distress about having the phobia.

F. The fear, anxiety or avoidance is persistent, typically lasting six or more months.

G. The fear or avoidance is not due to direct physiological effects of a substance (e.g., drugs, medications) or a general medical condition not better accounted for by another mental disorder.

Talking to your child

You now have some understanding of the signs and symptoms you can look out for in your child if you are concerned they are struggling with social anxiety. However, identifying signs can be quite difficult at times and your child might have developed some excellent strategies and excuses for avoiding particular situations.

You may also feel that this is simply 'part of who they are', but it is important to take into consideration how these difficulties will impact their ability to develop in the future when they are expected to attend college, university, move out of the family home or begin their career.

Because of this, it's important that these suspected – or clearly identified – problems with social anxiety are discussed with your child.

Not only will this help you gain a better understanding of what your child is experiencing, but it will also make them aware that you have noticed these difficulties, that you care about their experiences and that their difficulties can be normalized so they can be made aware they are not alone in experiencing these symptoms. Most importantly, they can be made aware that treatment is available for this type of problem.

To help think about your child and their experiences, when talking with them, it can be helpful to think of the 5Ws: What, When, Where, Why and Who with.

The 5Ws

What: What do they experience – feeling very anxious, very low, negative thoughts about themselves, feeling people judge them, feeling very lonely?

When: When do these feelings and experiences take place? Are they present all the time, or at particular times?

Where: Where do these experiences take place and where do they experience these symptoms of anxiety? This could be prior, during and following social interactions.

Why: Do they feel like they are likely to make a mistake in social situations, do they feel as though they are going to be judged negatively?

Who with: Do these experiences take place when they are on their own, with family, friends, and extended family or with a particular age group or people?

What to do as a parent

What we do know about social anxiety is that the first line of treatment should come in the form of CBT (Cognitive Behavioural Therapy). Evidence has shown us that other forms of treatment, including self-help, counselling, group therapy and medications are not as effective with social anxiety as they are in other difficulties, such as low mood.

Based on this information, I would always look to make a referral to your local CAMHS team if you suspect your child is presenting with social anxiety difficulties. Hopefully the information provided previously can help you share relevant information to these services, to enable them to accept your referral and begin working with your child.

We know that, unfortunately, child and adolescent services are not always able to see children immediately and at times there could be some wait to access therapy. The rest of this chapter offers some strategies and suggestions that can be implemented prior to accessing any help.

Set goals

Have your child choose realistic goals. A goal can help a child to think about what they want to achieve and allow them to have something to work towards in the here and now. It is also useful to think about a goal related to their future, as this will provide motivation, and a reason to achieve some of the more difficult goals that they might be setting themselves in the here and now.

An important part of setting short-term goals is to ensure that they are realistic, relevant to what they want to achieve, achievable in a timely manner and measurable, so you are both aware of when this has been achieved. It can also be nice to have at least three different goals that you will work towards.

It is a good idea to set one goal which might be achieved quite quickly to help provide a sense of accomplishment and movement, while the second goal might be one which you work towards over many months, and the third might be a long-term goal of your child's. By working backwards and thinking about your child's long-term goals (do they want to be a footballer? a scientist? a musician? a builder? an athlete? do they want to attend university?) you can both consider what they need to work on in the short term, and set some shorter and medium-term goals.

Initially agreeing short-term goals with your child will enable them to notice when they have achieved them. Allowing them to reach these goals will hopefully be helpful in giving them a sense of achievement. It is also useful to review any goals that you set with your child to see how they are managing in achieving what you have both set out to do. If a particular goal seems a little more difficult than expected, then it might be worthwhile breaking the steps down even further. For example, if a short-term goal was to speak to a new person in school but your child has struggled with this, you could break it down into smaller goals and simply set a new goal to smile at a new person, to make eye contact with them or to sit next to them in class. With this, the goals are more achievable but also link really well into their initial goal to speak to someone new in school.

Examples
Short-term goal: speak with the cashier in the local shop, talk to the postman, ask for directions from a stranger.
Medium-term goal: join a new club, start a new relationship with at least one person, meet a friend outside school once a week.
Long-term goal: set up my own clothes shop, become an actor, work with computer games, become a mechanic.

Working on what they do (their safety behaviours)
As we've already seen, some of a child's behaviours during social interactions may actually be contributing to their anxiety and making them stand out more, while also preventing them from challenging or disproving some of their negative thoughts.

A child with social anxiety may even feel these behaviours are helpful, and might be unwilling to stop using them – they may report that such 'safety behaviours' provide some relief from their anxiety.

To help with this, a useful strategy can be to write down all of the things they might do during social interactions to help their anxiety, but which in fact have a negative impact not only on their anxiety but also on their social interactions. Such things might include avoiding eye contact, rehearsing exactly what they are going to say, looking at the floor, putting headphones in their ears, covering their face, not talking, and so on.

To test out how helpful – or not – these behaviours are, you could set up an experiment with them. Set out an agreement with your child to enter a social interaction using their 'helpful' strategies as much as possible, while focusing all their attention on themselves and how anxious they feel. The interaction could be with yourself, a different relative or a friend of yours. No time limit needs to be attached to this, but it would be useful to try it for at least a few minutes.

Once it's finished, ask your child to do the complete opposite of what they were doing, avoiding the use of any of 'safety behaviours'. Instead, they should make eye contact, interact with the other person, keep their head up, uncover their face and focus their attention on the other person.

To help with learning in this experiment, it can be helpful to get your child to make predictions of what they think will happen in each scenario when they use their safety behaviours, and when they do not. This can include how anxious they feel they will be in each exercise (0 – not anxious, 10 – very anxious), how bad their negative thoughts will be (0 – not very bad, 10 – very bad), how comfortable the other person will feel in the interaction (0 – not at all, 10 – very comfortable) and how self-conscious they felt (0 – not at all, 10 –very self-conscious).

Once the exercise has been done, you can review the predictions, and think about the actual ratings after the interaction. Feedback can also be provided by the other person involved in this brief experiment.

The ratings should demonstrate a reduction in scores when not using safety behaviours. If this is not the case, it might be useful to try this exercise again with a different person, and for your child to increase their safety behaviours, exaggerating them as much as possible. This will really help test out how helpful they feel these behaviours are, if the initial exercise didn't quite work.

Exposing your child to social situations

The natural reaction of a parent is to help protect and shelter their child when they are anxious. Although this is a very tempting approach, what we know about anxiety is that if we continue to avoid it, it will not improve and can become more problematic over time.

By protecting and sheltering your child, you are unintentionally sending a message to them that there are dangers, risks and concerns from which they need protection.

To overcome this, it is important to provide them with confidence-building experiences, and to help reduce their avoidance of situations that make them anxious.

Gradual exposure is a useful tool for helping your child expose themselves to new social experiences. The idea behind it is to start small with social interactions that might not generate unmanageable amounts of anxiety, and to gradually increase these social interactions over time.

Once they begin to feel comfortable with a particular exercise within this exposure, they can then move on to the next social exercise which may generate more anxiety. It's important to remember that a child's anxiety may not always decrease completely, so once their anxiety reduces from a 10 to a 3, or a 4, when initiating this social interaction (10 – feeling very anxious, 0 – not anxious at all) then it is probably a good time to move on to the next task.

Gradual exposure to new social experiences will help your child build much needed social skills and increase their confidence in their own abilities. This gradual exposure might be difficult and will most likely require some pressure from you as a parent, but it is important that your child is involved in agreeing to this gradual exposure and you can think together about the steps they will take. (An example of an exposure ladder can be found in Chapter 3.)

Remember, work to their strengths and involve them in interactions where they might feel more comfortable. They might have interests in video games, animals, sports or other things, so think about using these interests to their advantage and incorporate them in the exposure work and within their goals.

Focusing on the positives

What we know about people who experience social anxiety is that they will often focus on the negatives in the social inter- action and their physical experiences of their anxiety symptoms. For a child, this may be about how they feel about themselves, such as weird or stupid, or it could be concentrating on negative things that they feel have happened, such as tripping over a word, shaking, not being able to look others in the eye. As a result, they will often miss out on all the positive experiences they might have had during the interaction.

With this in mind, it can be useful to set a task and to get your child to focus on these positives. Set up an experiment together, perhaps during the course of a day in school, or during a single visit to a shop, for example.

The idea is to get your child to focus on all the positive things that take place during these interactions. This might include the other person talking back to them, smiling, making eye contact, asking them a question, wanting to know more about them, asking how they are, and so on.

Once these positives have been identified, it can be useful to write them down on a piece of paper so you and they can remember them as facts for later on. Writing them down helps to:

1 Captures this information, as it can often be forgotten.
2 Reduces the focus on all of the negative aspects that the child believes may have taken place if they are dwelling on social interactions.

Managing worry before social interactions

This is a problem that often prevents children from engaging in social interactions. They are often predicting what might happen prior to anything actually taking place, predicting the future in a way which is not possible.

It can be helpful to question your child on how they know what will happen in future social interactions. Referring to previous work relating to 'thinking errors' could be particularly helpful, as predicting the future is not possible and it is likely that they are falling into this thinking trap.

Another helpful strategy to use would be to think about the pros and cons of engaging in this type of thinking. You can write this information down together, in the hope of identifying that thinking about all the negative possible outcomes has very little benefit, as these predictions are often inaccurate and fail to provide a picture of how the actual situations will turn out.

A child may also ask what might happen, or what if particular problems happen, while also seeking reassurance about the outcome. It can be difficult not to engage in these conversations and not to provide the reassurance that nothing bad will happen. Unfortunately, we simply don't know this will be the case, so you may find it helpful to respond in a different manner. You could ask your child:

What are the possible outcomes?
What happened last time?
Because that happened last time, does it mean it will happen again?
How will we find out this is true, or not true?

This will help allow your child to think more independently about what might happen and help them develop their own strategies for managing future situations, whether these are social ones or not.

Modelling helpful behaviour

Modelling helpful behaviour in front of your child is a further helpful strategy that can be applied. It could be that you also struggle in social situations or that you avoid potential social interactions where possible.

Even if this is not the case, it is good to model helpful behaviour and possibly to demonstrate to your child how you overcome your own anxieties (Chapter 2 offers some more information on modelling).

How you do this will depend on you and your child. It could be that you also struggle with social anxieties and, if this is the case, it might be that you set similar goals with your child. By doing this, you will demonstrate to your child that you too are willing to work on something that is very difficult, so they become aware that it is possible to overcome anxieties and engage in activities that you could not have done previously.

It might also mean that you need further support initially in overcoming these difficulties. If this is the case, great – it shows that seeking further support is acceptable and perfectly normal. Hopefully it will also help demonstrate, after you've accessed help, that therapy can be useful.

If you don't experience social anxiety, this is also fine, and different goals can be set. It might be that you have a specific phobia of dogs, spiders or small spaces. If this is the case, then you can demonstrate your willingness to overcome these fears and let your child observe not just your intention to overcome, but more importantly how you actually manage and face those anxieties.

Callum

Callum is an 11-year-old boy who has recently moved from primary to secondary school. His dad has a history of anxiety and Callum has always appeared a little anxious to his parents, but they have managed this quite well by protecting him from his anxieties and ensuring he attended a very small primary school in their local village which had very small classrooms and a close network of teachers.

Callum appeared to settle quite well into secondary school but, as previous peers began to form their own groups, Callum struggled to make new friends and began to report that particular students would bully and mock him during lunch breaks. This was short-lived and quickly resolved by the school; however, at a similar time, when one of his teachers asked Callum to stand and read aloud in front of his peers, he made some minor mistakes, which resulted in his classmates laughing at him.

After this incident in school Callum began to minimize his interactions in each class. He would no longer put his hand up, would avoid eye contact with the teacher and his peers, and he had thoughts that people would judge and laugh at him if he made a mistake when talking to a classmate or answering a question. He began to minimize time with the few friends he had in school and spent more time alone during lunch breaks in the library where he would sit and read, or spend time on a computer.

At the same time his parents saw that his mood appeared much lower during the school week, and on Sunday evenings his sleep began to become a problem. He became more anxious and reluctant to attend shops where people of a similar age might be present, and he appeared visibly anxious in the mornings when attending school – but he continued to attend and his attendance remained very good.

Callum did appear much brighter in mood on a Friday evening and during the weekend. However, his social interactions with others outside of the family were limited as he felt much more comfortable at home, though he would speak with some friends online while playing games.

Think about Callum's situation and try and answer the following questions:

- What could have made Callum more susceptible to anxiety?
- Which events do you feel contributed to his anxiety symptoms in social situations?
- Is it helpful for Callum to continue to avoid putting his hand up and reducing his verbal interactions with his peers?
- Why does Callum's mood appear to become brighter on the weekend?

Now think about the strategies provided in this chapter. What could Callum's parents do to help him? Should they continue to help him avoid his anxieties? Try completing an exposure ladder for Callum to move forward with his difficulties. This exercise will help you apply some of the helpful strategies and learning that you have read here, which you can also use with your own child to support their social anxiety difficulties.

References and further reading

American Psychiatric Association (2013) *Diagnostic and Statistical Manual of Mental Disorders (5th Edition): DSM-V* Washington, DC: American Psychiatric Association.

NHS Digital (2017) Mental Health of Children and Young People in England, 2017. [Online]. Available at: <digital.nhs.uk/data-and-information/publications/statistical/mental-health-of-children-and-young-people-in-england/2017/2017> (accessed: 9 June 2020).

8

Worries about being away from others

Dr Kristina Keeley-Jones, Clinical Psychologist

Being with – and feeling safely connected to – our caregiver and attachment figure when we are growing as a child is a primal human need (Bowlby, 2005), a need that often stays with us even into adulthood. The strong and persistent bonds we develop with our children leave them with templates for their own future, and help them to understand themselves, other people and the world around them. These templates will later influence how our children connect and bond with their own children and shape the generations thereafter.

Given our attachment figure can provide a sense of safety and comfort, it is understandable that being away from those who we are connected to the most can be an unsettling time for anyone, let alone a child. Our children are frequently faced with new challenges and experiences such as starting nursery, moving schools, trying a new hobby, or being away from home for a school trip or a friend's sleepover.

Feeling worried about being away from others or from the familiarity and comfort of home is often a natural feature of child development and of growing up. Nevertheless, parenting a child in distress can often be upsetting, unsettling and frustrating, especially when as parents we want to try and help to make things better for our children. (I am using the words 'parenting' and 'parent' to describe the actions of people who perform the active role of caregiver for a child).

This chapter aims to provide some comfort, understanding and security when everyone's feelings are running high and strong, and the way forward seems uncertain.

How to spot attachment worries

Evie
Evie had always been a 'difficult' child who had been hard to soothe and calm down. Parenting her was often overwhelming and exhausting, so when she started screaming and crying at her parents not to leave her at nursery it all felt too much. It was horrible to see Evie in such an emotional mess, and the panic in her eyes (and sometimes red-faced rage) when her parents had to say goodbye at nursery punched a wave of fear, sadness and guilt in their stomachs when they tried to leave. It was a battle getting her out of the house every morning. Life felt hard.

The struggles for Evie and her parents may be familiar to many parents who have had to leave a child in the care of others. Just as Evie's vocal protests of separation are indicators of her levels of distress, there may also be other signs that a child might be struggling with worries about being away from you, such as:

- Dawdling or 'naughty' behaviours that get you sucked in to extending the time you are with them.
- Emotional outbursts of anger or rage.
- Nightmares with themes about worries of being away from others, being abandoned, getting lost, or being alone.
- Excessive crying, seeming inconsolable, clinging to you.
- Physical symptoms such as tummy upsets, headaches, muscle pains that have no medical cause.
- Refusing to leave your home.
- Worrying that you will not come back or that something bad will happen.
- Worrying they won't manage without you being there.

The above is a brief list of some of the types of behaviours and emotions that children may show us when they are worried about being away from us. There may also be other signs that you have noticed that indicate that your child is struggling and it is important to listen to yourself and make a note of these as you will know your child best.

What can make worries grow stronger?

Parenting a child who finds it hard to embrace new situations, people or challenges can make us feel overwhelmed, frustrated or frozen with uncertainty. When we imagine being a parent, most of us never imagine just how much our children's emotional displays can awaken our own hidden – and often raw – emotions. Not knowing how to respond to our child can make us feel anxious and helpless, or we might feel that nothing works, leaving us at a loss about what to do next.

Thinking about what is going on for your child, yourself or other family members is one of the ways in which we can start to understand and help your child manage their distress. If we can stop for a moment and think about our current situation and what is happening in our own and our children's lives, there may be clues that can be used as the first stepping stones towards building an understanding of how to strengthen feelings of comfort and security for your child.

Life events and change can unsettle the most confident children and families. If there has been recent loss or bereavement, including the loss of a pet, a home move, or another stressor that has caused everyone to feel unsettled, it can sometimes make sense that your child might be clingier, reluctant to leave you, or struggle with worries about separation. Other things that can often unsettle children include:

- Illness.
- Traumatic incidents such as accidents, social unrest.
- Family distress.
- Changes or inconsistencies in daily routines or parenting.
- Parental absence.
- Feeling uncertain if and when a parent will return.
- School changes, difficulties at school.
- Impending or recent transition to a new school.
- Separations, divorce, births and other family changes such as a parent's loss of their job.

At other times, we may struggle to find any clarity around what has made a situation feel so difficult for our child. At these times we may have to take a little more time to discover and make guesses about what our children's underlying needs could be. This is not always easy, but by thinking about our child and putting ourselves in their shoes, we can begin to see things differently. When we see things differently, we can start to make the changes that are sometimes necessary to support our child.

What you can do to help

As a parent it is not always easy to know how to help. However, there are a number of small changes that you can make to help you understand and manage your child's worries and distress.

Spot, think and link

Firstly, if we can develop a better understanding of anxiety and worry, including the effects of anxiety on our bodies including the fight, flight and freeze responses (see Chapter 1 for more detail), we can increase our awareness of and sensitivity to the signs of our child's responses to worry.

Developing your awareness and sensitivity towards your child can help you notice your child's struggles and challenges, and this will enable you to better identify the things that may be helpful to calm them down at that moment. It is important that this increased awareness and sensitivity is not intrusive for your child, so it is usually more helpful to keep these initial observations and thoughts about them to yourself. You may also find it helpful to share them with another supportive adult at a time when your child cannot hear these conversations. If a child frequently hears an adult talk to others about all the things that are challenging the child it can lead children to feel more self-conscious and anxious about their difficulties.

Imagine your child is becoming more and more anxious about having to leave you but they are not quite at the stage of childhood development where they are able to notice or speak about their body clues and bubbling discomfort. Being able to spot some of these signs of worry (for example, fidgeting, running around, flitting from topic to topic, forgetting what you have said, having sweaty hands, or perhaps another sign) will be important in shaping the way you think about and respond to their emotional needs.

Hassan

Whenever it was a school morning, Hassan was always doing the opposite to what his parents asked. He whined and complained when told to get dressed into his school uniform and endlessly provoked his brother by calling him names. Hassan often refused to get dressed and so his Mum would end up helping him. Hassan often threw his shoes at the door when he had to get them on, and would then run and hide when they had to leave the house, often making everyone late. When they got to school, Hassan would become very quiet and tell his Mum he had to go home as he was sick.

Given Hassan's behaviours are quite obviously and significantly disruptive to his family's morning routine, it probably wouldn't be that difficult to spot that Hassan was finding something difficult. The harder part for some parents can be figuring out the underlying hidden emotional needs that a child's behaviours may be communicating. It would be easy to assume that Hassan was being 'naughty' or 'mean', or for his parents and brother to blame him for creating problems in the family, or for family members to shout and fight back at Hassan, or think he had some underlying disorder that needed a diagnosis.

Fortunately, Hassan's parents had been able to make space in their busy lives to spend time calmly talking and reflecting about the changes in his behaviours that they had spotted over the past few months. They remembered that Hassan had told them about another child at school who had been calling him names, and that his grandmother had experienced a recent fall which had upset him. Being able to think together and make guesses about what may be making Hassan feel worried about being away from others enabled his parents to link these worries about school and his grandmother to his unsettled behaviours at home.

As we can see from the experiences of Hassan and his family, spotting obvious or more hidden signs of worry and anxiety in your child, thinking about what may be happening in your child's life and linking these together are important stages that will help you to begin to provide the right support for your child. We will consider other ways to help your child feel more secure and connected later in this chapter.

Thinking about your child and their hidden needs

As well as providing comfort, nurture, guidance and acceptable limits, parenting is a bit like a detective. Anyone who has held a writhing and squawking baby will have likely encountered momentary anxiety about not knowing what they want or need. We may change a nappy, offer a feed or try to rock the baby to sleep in a process of elimination until something works to calm them. As children grow, their needs change and layers of complexity build, but it is still important to try to understand what is going on for our children. It is also absolutely crucial that we can recognize that our children's physical, social and emotional needs are different and separate to that of our own.

Spot, think, link and label

As discussed earlier, being able to spot signs of distress, think about what may be happening for our child and link these together can help us to understand what is underlying our child's behaviours or emotions. This greater understanding can lead us to be able to support in ways that may help your child feel more secure and connected, and these feelings of security and connection may reduce the levels of worry and anxiety that your child may be experiencing. It can be helpful to think of the metaphor of our child's more overt behaviours and emotions being the tip of the iceberg, with the parts of the iceberg that are underwater representing our child's hidden emotional experiences and needs (see Chapter 3).

Stopping what you are doing, putting down your phone or turning off the television, and turning your attention to your child and really listening to what they are saying with their words and their bodies can help you see what may be churning around in the water under the iceberg of emotions.

Sitting with your child, listening and being emotionally available (without getting upset yourself) when they experience the worry feelings can show your child that you are able to manage these feelings, and that these feelings do not worry or overwhelm you. This may help them to understand that big strong feelings can be survived and, importantly, that these feelings will eventually change over time.

When we are able to make a guess about how our children may be feeling by listening and 'tuning in' to our child using our sensitivity and empathy, we can then more easily connect with our child's emotional world and name the emotion they may be experiencing. Labelling our children's emotions can often help to tame the emotions (Siegel and Bryson, 2012) and the intensity of the emotion will reduce over time. The experience of having our emotions listened to and understood by another person is one of the most powerful ways to feel connected to, validated and soothed by another human being.

What gets in the way of being able to spot, think, link and label?

Distractions such as work, the daily tasks of life, and endless chores can get in the way of us being physically and emotionally available to our child. When we are more distracted and disconnected it is understandable that we will be less sensitive and able to spot what might be going on for our child. The pressures that come with being an adult and a parent can sometimes crowd out or overpower our ability to think about our child. Sometimes, our own past experiences may muddle how we view our child or their responses to their own experiences.

It is expected that there will be times when our ability to focus on our child's needs *will* become disrupted, and it is important to be kind to ourselves when this inevitably happens. Being aware of these disruptions means we can then repair our emotional connection with our child.

Other things that are important for us to be aware of when helping our child with worries include: calming our emotions down first before responding to our child (see Chapter 2 for more ideas on how to do this); seeking out social support; noticing our own reactions to our child's behaviours and emotions; and understanding our own history of being parented.

Noticing your own emotional reaction to the worries

When supporting your child with their distress in being away from others, it will be important to be aware of your own reactions to their distress. By recognizing your own thoughts and emotions that are being triggered by your child's worries, this will help sort out the emotions that belong to your child and the emotions that belong to you.

Some of the common parental responses include:

Worry: 'What if they never manage to leave me without getting so upset?'

Fear: 'I don't know what to do, I've lost control.'

Guilt: 'I've passed on my own worries to them. What have I done to make them like this?'

Shame: 'How embarrassing that they're clinging to me like this. What will others think?'

Anger and frustration: 'Why won't they just go and have fun?'

By noticing and being aware of your own thoughts and reactions, you will then be more able to respond to your child's distress in a meaningful way.

Understanding your own history and emotions

No matter how much we might try and shelter our children, they often pick up on the emotions of others around them, so if we worry, our children may worry too.

If you find yourself to be a worrier (and most of us are at times), then the best present that you can give to your child is for you to spend some time focussing on learning ways to manage your own worry. This will help you to keep calm when your child is distressed.

When our children become very distressed, we might find that this is overwhelming and difficult to tolerate. How we respond in the present is often shaped by our past, and we all have our own unique experiences of being parented. Sometimes these past experiences continue to influence the way we manage emotions and respond in our current relationships (Van der Kolk, 2014), including the relationships with our children.

You may have already benefited from emotional support in the form of therapy or counselling in order to help make sense of your past experiences. If so, by being aware of your past, learning how to manage your emotions, and being active in getting support when needed, you will be in a wonderfully strong position to effectively help your child.

Other strategies to support children who worry about being away from others

Once we understand some of the reasons that might be underlying a child's worries about being away from others, we can support them more effectively.

Your child may need you to connect with nursery or school to get additional support or nurture for them. Other areas that might need to be strengthened for your child include increasing their sense of safety in others and the world, and building their own sense of mastery and competence in understanding and managing their worries.

Increasing your child's sense of safety and trust in others and the world

Thinking about what makes your child feel safe and reintroducing those things in your relationship can help increase their feelings of security and connectedness to you. Some parents find it helpful to reconnect though playing games that increase positive emotions, talking about comforting family memories, providing additional nurture, and ensuring stability and consistency through family routines and parenting approaches.

William

William used to be such a happy baby who 'was no trouble at all', so it didn't make sense to his parents why he had suddenly turned into such a clingy child. William's dad, Joe, thought he needed to toughen William up and would tell him that he had nothing to be upset about. Nothing his parents did helped, and William would just hide and freeze behind his parents' arms and beg them not to leave him. Joe had always liked school and after-school groups so he wanted William to have the same experiences as him. He felt embarrassed by William and wanted him to be like a 'normal' child.

Think about how things might be different for William if Joe is able to connect with William as well as acknowledge his own feelings of shame, embarrassment and uncertainty that have been awoken through parenting his son. Consider what it would feel like for William if Joe were to validate how it can feel unsettling getting used to new experiences like school, and to hear Joe's soothing words saying that he would be able to help support William through these tricky feelings of worry.

Validating emotions can be a powerful way of helping your child feel heard and connected to you. Remember, it is okay to validate your child's emotional reactions, even if you do not agree with their viewpoint. The principle that you are supporting your child with is that it is okay to feel how they do given that this is an emotional experience that is unique to them. It is also not the same as validating that they are right to be worried about being away from you.

It can be tricky to work out what validating and invalidating statements are. Below are examples of each to help make this clearer:

Invalidating statement: 'You may not like going to school, but at least your school is a good one! Lots of other children don't even get a nice school to go to.'

Validating statement: 'It seems like you're having a tough time going to school at the moment. It is understandable you're finding it tricky – everything is so new and you are still finding out where to go and who your teachers are. Let's sit down together and let me help you figure things out.'

In addition to validating your child's experiences, you can further strengthen your connections with your child and build your child's feelings of safety by providing acceptance of your child with empathy (Golding and Hughes, 2012).

Children thrive when they are thought about with kindness by their parents. You can make them aware you are thinking about them even when you aren't around, for example, by writing loving notes to be found in their lunchboxes, or if they are older, they may like to discover sticky notes in surprising places detailing the tangible things you love about them. You will need to tailor this to the age of the child as not many teenagers would want friends to see these notes!

Importantly, try not to make unrealistic promises. We cannot completely get rid of worry, nor can we prevent every situation that causes worry. What we can do is to be there for them, connect with them and support them to manage the worries.

Building your child's sense of mastery and competence

It is usually helpful if we can normalize our children's experience of emotions. Having worries and other uncomfortable feelings is to be expected and is a part of normal human existence. It can be helpful when we gently celebrate and remind our child of other times where they managed to tolerate a situation and get through it even when their worries were very strong. This will slowly help increase our child's tolerance to other distressing emotions.

Additional strategies that can help include:

- Setting boundaries around how many kisses or hugs will be given when you say goodbye.
- Focusing on what positive things will happen when they are away from you.
- Telling them you are going as sneaking off can make things worse.
- Telling them when you are coming back and that you look forward to hearing all about their day when you pick them up.
- Ensuring you don't avoid a situation due to their worry – avoiding will likely make things trickier in the long run. Small steps in exposure will give opportunities for your child to learn to tolerate these uncomfortable feelings (see Chapter 7 for more ideas around understanding exposure).
- Making guesses and helping them label their feelings.
- Playing calming and soothing music if you are travelling by car can help. It is usually more helpful to decide together what type of music you will play when you are both calm and connected in the relationship.
- Making sure your child has your full attention when you reunite with them. Imagine if you were to meet a friend after

a long time and they were constantly preoccupied on their phone or not really listening to you, it would most likely not feel very nice and would not make you feel secure or valued in the relationship. The same is true for children.

• Asking for help from people who are supportive when it is getting too much.
• Increasing your levels of emotional availability during the time you spend with your child – including spending time playing together.

Externalize worry

Separating out a problem from the person (also known as externalizing the problem; White, 2007) can be a helpful strategy when supporting children to manage emotional challenges. Being able to talk with your child about how 'the worry' or 'the worrysaurus' might be stopping your child from joining in with activities they usually enjoy can help to reduce the likelihood of your child experiencing themselves as bad or shameful.

Soothing strategy ideas

Soothing with the senses (also discussed in Chapter 12) can be a great way of calming strong emotions. Think about trying out essential oils, herbs and spices from your cupboard, hand lotions, slime or 'gloop' (cornflour and water), Play-Doh, chewy sweets, popping candy, a small piece of chocolate, bouncing on a gym ball, calming music, soft or furry fabrics, two-way sequins, nice photos of nature scenes and listening to nature sounds or calming music.

Using your child's imagination can be a great way of helping them regulate their breathing, for example getting them to exhale for six seconds when blowing up an imaginary balloon or blowing a real or imaginary feather. Helping children slow their breathing can be an effective way of calming down emotions, and blowing bubbles or using their teddy to rest on their tummy while they slowly breathe in and out can be a fun and calming way to help your child feel soothed.

It is important to practise using different soothing strategies when your child is calm and willing. It will help to keep things fun and playful and let your child lead on what they like and don't like. Making time to explore what helps your child can be a fun and enjoyable task for both of you, and you may even find some things that help you feel calm too!

References and further reading

Bowlby, J. (2005) *The Making and Breaking of Affectional Bonds*. London: Routledge.

Golding, K. and Hughes, D. (2012) *Creating Loving Attachments*. London: Jessica Kingsley Publishers.

Siegel, D.J. and Bryson, T.P. (2012) *The Whole-Brain Child: 12 Proven Strategies to Nurture Your Child's Developing Mind*. London: Constable & Robinson Ltd.

Van der Kolk, B.A. (2014) *The Body Keeps the Score: Brain, Mind, and Body in the Healing of Trauma*. New York: Viking.

White, M. (2007) *Maps of Narrative Practice*. New York: Norton Books.

9

Obsessions and compulsions

Sam Thompson, RMN & CBT Therapist

This chapter looks at obsessions and compulsions and identifies how they present in children. We will look at the different types of compulsions and obsessions and how they are maintained as a problem, including body dysmorphia. The chapter ends with some simple techniques to help overcome obsessions and compulsions.

What is OCD and how may it affect my child?

Obsessive Compulsive Disorder (often referred to as OCD) can have a significant impact on the lives of children and their families. Research shows that OCD behaviours can interfere with academic, social and home functioning (Allsopp and Verduyn, 1989). If your child is struggling with OCD, you can help them by gaining a greater understanding of what OCD is.

OCD is often defined by two aspects: obsessional thoughts and compulsions. Intrusive thoughts/images can cause a child significant stress and worry; some children experiencing these obsessional thoughts may feel the need to carry out a 'compulsion' as a way to temporarily reduce the distress they are experiencing. The compulsions that your child has may not be obvious to everyone. Outlined in the section below are the most common obsessional thoughts and compulsions among children.

Obsessional thoughts

Obsessional thoughts relate to children experiencing a recurrent and persistent thought or image that is often difficult to displace. We all experience intrusive thoughts; it is relatively common. For example, you are standing on the kerbside waiting to cross a busy road when suddenly you think: 'If I stepped in front of that traffic right now, I'd be squashed flat'. The thought pops into your mind and leaves your short-term memory in a similar fashion. You may have completely forgotten about the incident while you were on your walk. However, someone who experiences intrusive thoughts will find that the image or the experience constantly reappears in their mind. The constant reappearance of intrusive thoughts provokes anguish, distress and upset for a child. When the obsessional thought is experienced, your child will try to do anything to remove the image from their mind as quickly as possible to ease the distress. One of the closest examples I can give would be imagining a nightmare that you once had where the images were so vivid that they felt real. Now, imagine this nightmare is played on repeat, all day, every day. This is how it feels to experience obsessional thoughts.

The thought or image that your child is experiencing may be particularly anxiety provoking and distressing – but you should be aware that their worries with obsessional thinking may not always relate to real-life problems, as you'll see from the list of the most common types of thoughts, below:

- **Fear of contamination:** Your child may have a fear of being contaminated by someone or something. They may also worry about falling ill from either a virus, germs or dirt. This may cause your child to avoid any potential contamination due to fear of being ill and potentially dying, resulting in extra precautions to reduce the chances of this happening, such as excess hand-washing, multiple showers or even insisting that their clothing is washed every day.
- **Fear of harm:** Your child may have a fear of themselves or others coming to harm. Experiencing these thoughts may mean that he or she feels a sense of guilt or responsibility simply for thinking that something bad could happen to someone that they know and love.
- **Thoughts of harm/violence:** Your child may experience thoughts of wanting to hurt themselves or other people. This can lead them to feeling that they are a danger to others, and that people won't like them, or will judge them. Having these recurring thoughts can lead your child to become more

isolated from their peer group and family members. When children get these thoughts, it doesn't mean that they are going to hurt themselves or others. It is important to separate the thought from the action.

- **Religious thoughts:** Your child may be experiencing thoughts relating to religion and feeling anxious about not following certain aspects from a religious book such as the Bible, or following routine prayers. He or she may feel worried about upsetting and offending God.

Compulsions

If a young person is experiencing obsessional thoughts that are causing them anxiety and distress then they may feel the need to find a way to reduce this. If we feel anxious or upset as human beings then we always look at ways of trying to manage these feelings. No one likes to be anxious or distressed. A child experiencing intrusive thoughts may look to reduce them by carrying out a compulsion. A compulsion describes a repetitive form of behaviour that the child carries out to reduce their levels of distress. Shown below are some of the many common examples of compulsions that you may – or may not – have noticed in your child. This isn't a definitive list and there may be other compulsions that the child carries out – they may even be unaware of them until they talk about their worries:

- **Hand washing:** Washing hands an excessive amount of times and for a prolonged period of time. You may notice your child wash their hands once and then continue to do so several times in a subsequent fashion. There might be occasions where children will feel the need to constantly clean and disinfect surfaces in their bedroom or when using school toilets and lockers.
- **Ordering:** Placing objects in their bedroom in a certain way, not wanting any objects to be removed from their bedroom or making sure that they do not allow family or friends to touch parts of their room. You may notice your child become upset if their bedroom has been cleaned, or certain objects taken away.
- **Repeating:** The child may have to repeat certain words or behaviours to themselves, sometimes this is without anyone

else hearing or knowing. They may feel that the words or behaviours need to be completed in a certain order and must be carried out in that fashion. Any disruption or break in the sequence can cause greater distress for the child.

- **Checking:** Relates to ensuring that something is turned on or off in the house. Common examples for young people include checking that light switches or bath taps are turned off in the house. They may also repeatedly check that their charger or hair straighteners have been turned off at the switch. Children may also seek reassurance from friends and family about this (see Chapter 1 for more information about reassurance).
- **Counting:** These compulsions relate to a behaviour being completed for a specific number of times. For example, they may check the light switch has been turned off four times. Your child may count to certain numbers or sequence of numbers in their head without other people noticing.

Body dysmorphic disorder (BDD)

You may notice your child make reference to their physical features, and on how such features appear to others. They may discuss features of their face or body that they don't particularly find appealing, and may be self-critical. This can lead to further preoccupations about their physical appearance and how it presents to others. Children may feel the need to check parts of their face numerous times during the day, often looking in the mirror and highlighting features of themselves. There is a tendency for there to be an overlap with children experiencing body dysmorphic disorder (BDD) and eating disorders. However, it is worth highlighting that BDD tends to focus on a specific body part which may not be visible to others, whereas children with eating disorders are preoccupied by their overall body image, weight or size.

Strategies

As parents you will want to know how to support your child properly, which is why we have outlined the following strategies to help encourage this. If you have any doubts or you are unsure about them then please contact your local CAMHS clinician who will be able to guide you.

Understanding how anxiety works

Higher levels of anxiety can have a significant impact on OCD, especially with the intrusive thoughts and compulsions your child may experience. Return to Chapter 1 to learn about anxiety and how it is experienced in the body and mind. If your child is experiencing greater levels of anxiety then they may experience greater intrusive thoughts and compulsions.

Be curious

If your teenager is experiencing obsessional thoughts and carrying out compulsions of any kind, it will be distressing and upsetting not only for them, but also for you and other members in your family. Younger children may be blissfully unaware of what's happening, but they are incredibly susceptible to picking up on distress and upset from their siblings. It is important to leave emotions 'at the door', especially with regard to your own feelings. For someone experiencing compulsions and obsessional thoughts, if it was that simple to treat, then no one would develop them. Instead, adopt a 'curious' approach, especially when talking to your child. Imagine an old-fashioned detective with a magnifying glass, searching for clues. We need to know why the young person is feeling upset or angry. For example, you can say:

> 'Can you tell me how you're feeling?'
> 'What's happening?'
> 'I've noticed you've been washing your hands a lot more recently. Is everything okay? Can you talk to me about what's going on?'

Reassurance seeking

If your child is feeling anxious and experiencing obsessions and compulsions, they may have a tendency to seek reassurance from you or someone else they know. This is often known as 'reassurance seeking' and a child will resort to it to help them to ease their anxieties quickly. Paradoxically, frequent reassurance can have a detrimental impact on your child's well-being and may increase their urge to seek it from you (see Chapter 1). Your child may also insist on wanting to continue implementing the rituals triggered by their obsessional thoughts.

Abraham

Abraham is a 13-year-old boy who lives with both his parents and pet dog Mollie. Over the last couple of years, his parents have noticed that Abraham has been washing his hands more often than he should. His mother mentioned that it wasn't just before meal times, it was becoming more frequent, and they were having to replenish the hand wash every week. Abraham's father noticed that his hands were starting to look dry and cracked. When asked about this, Abraham would deny that there was a problem, often becoming angry at his parents. The family have noticed that Abraham would complete his daily tasks in a certain way, as well as checking that certain appliances were turned off, such as the oven and the phone charger under his bed.

Figure 9.1 shows an example of a frequent conversation that Abraham has with his mother. It shows how Abraham is feeling as he asks his mother for reassurance that his hands are indeed clean, despite washing them for a prolonged period of time. If Abraham receives this reassurance from his mother, it in fact – inadvertently – reinforces the feeling of worry for Abraham. This causes his potential worries to increase over time, and helps them develop into other situations, such as going out of the house and feeling worried that something in the house may not have been switched off. If Abraham's mother reduces reassurance, Abraham will have to reassure himself and this will improve his anxiety overall.

It's important to acknowledge that although providing reassurance isn't particularly helpful for your child, you should only reduce the amount of reassurance you give gradually over a period of time, going with what you feel comfortable with. There is a fine balance to be struck with the levels of reassurance given; if it is stopped immediately, it can cause further repercussions for your child. You may want to monitor how often your child asks

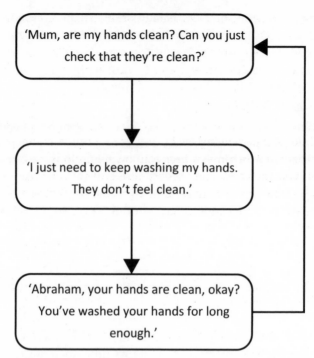

Figure 9.1 Reassurance seeking

you for reassurance during the day and record it on your mobile phone or on a piece of paper. When you have a rough number, you can then slowly reduce the amount of reassurance given, and encourage your child to recognize how they're feeling and what they can do to manage their anxiety.

Not letting OCD take control

Children who have OCD often describe how the obsessional thoughts and compulsions are taking control of their lives. One of the ways you can help your child to manage is to encourage them to 'fight back' against the OCD behaviours that are driving the feelings of worry and distress. Encouraging your child to take control of the OCD, instead of letting the OCD take control of them, is pivotal in improving the outcomes and will help to develop their confidence, especially as it can be common for a child with OCD symptoms to experience lower self-esteem. Externalizing your child's difficulty (see 'externalize the worry' strategy later in this chapter) can also help with this.

Choice of language

It is completely understandable to feel a range of emotions when your child is experiencing OCD. You are a human being and of course there may be times when your own emotions may get the better of you and cause you to react differently to how you would normally. However, it is important to recognize that the choice of language you use can also have an impact on your child who is experiencing OCD. Often, dismissing a child's experiences or displaying a consistently cynical attitude can have potentially damaging consequences. It can also make your child feel less validated, especially with the difficult experience they are having. Adjusting your approach to listen and recognize what your child is going through can lay the foundations for helping them to have the skills and confidence to overcome what is a distressing and upsetting time. Providing your child with the time and space to listen and understand what they're experiencing encourages them to open up about their difficulties. Often children are reluctant to discuss their difficulties for a variety of reasons, most notably the fear of being invalidated and judged, as well as being concerned about what others may think of them.

Neutralizing the thought

A child who experiences intrusive thoughts feels a high level of distress and upset and will often try to 'neutralize' these thoughts. 'Neutralizing' refers to the process of carrying out a compulsion to remove the intrusive thought or image. By doing this, your child temporarily reduces the levels of distress for a short period of time. However, the more they experience the intrusive thoughts or image, the more likely it is that they will continue to carry out the compulsions. Depending on the levels of anxiety and the distressing thoughts your child is experiencing, you may often see an increase in the compulsive acts, as your child uses their compulsions to 'prevent' their thoughts that something bad will happen or become true.

Have a conversation with your child about how they can alter the intrusive thoughts they are currently experiencing. Although discussing and explaining their thoughts may make them feel more anxious or upset, encourage alternative strategies such as balancing out the intrusive thought by exploring the positive memories and images that they have. Imagery can be incredibly powerful for children to use, especially when they let go and use their imagination. They may have a favourite memory, such as a holiday or family moment. Encourage them to explore this and to use these thoughts whenever they begin to feel anxious or upset. This skill can take time but will encourage your child to balance negative intrusive thoughts with alternative ways of thinking when confronting a situation. If that form of imagery does not seem to have an impact, then discuss ways of making the images 'sillier' or introduce something that may make your child laugh. Often encouraging young people to think about 'silly' images or something that they may find funny can help to reduce their levels of distress overall. Exploring other ways to manage the thoughts experienced can help to reduce the compulsions.

Write it down

When children are feeling particularly anxious or worried about a certain situation they tend to ruminate. Although we are not mind readers and don't claim to be, we can detect this from certain ways in which children act, especially when they're experiencing obsessions and compulsions. One way to help manage ruminations is to encourage the child to write down the worries they're experiencing in a table similar to the one below. The table encourages children to externalize their experiences when they've felt particularly worried. Each column breaks down the current situation into what was happening, as well as their thoughts and feelings around it. If writing it down on paper is difficult for the child, there are plenty of free accessible apps you can use, as well as using the tablet or computer to type up what they have been experiencing.

What was going on?	How it made me feel?	What I was thinking about?	What I did?
Didn't want to go back to school after the weekend.	Initially worried and stressed but relieved afterwards.	I didn't want anything bad to happen to my family.	I counted in my head in multiples of 3 to the number 30.

Figure 9.2 Example of a thought diary

Don't assume

It may be instinctive to want to assume what's going on for your child, especially if they're shy or reluctant to talk about it. For a child who is particularly worried, regardless of what the worry is, they need to be encouraged to share what is going on for them, in their own way. If we start to make assumptions about how a child is feeling, then they may feel that they can't share their worries or that what they're experiencing isn't important. Continue to encourage the child to express how they're feeling through other mediums, such as drawing, painting and using crafts. We all have different ways to express how we feel so it's important to understand and recognize that. The conversation may look something like this:

Parent: Kamal, I've noticed that you seem a bit worried. Is everything okay?

Kamal: I don't know how I feel.

Parent: That's okay, we don't always know how we're feeling at times. I know you're good at drawing so would you like to draw me a picture?

Kamal: Yeah, of course.

Parent: That's a really detailed drawing Kamal. What do these lines mean?

Kamal: These lines often mean I feel angry and upset.

Parent: Why do you feel angry and upset?

Kamal: I feel angry and upset when I think something bad will happen to us.

Externalize the worry

A child experiencing obsessional thinking and compulsions may feel hurt and upset if their behaviours are challenged by friends and family. They may take the comments personally and internalize them, causing further distress. It can also make them reluctant to want to talk about their worries or difficulties. One way to help young people talk about things is to externalize their behaviours and refer to them with a name of their choice. Giving compulsions a name can help young people to recognize what it is that they need to work towards and to overcome. Encourage your child to think of a name, and even to draw a picture, if they would like to. Often children will draw a monster to describe their thoughts and feelings towards the compulsions and obsessions they are experiencing. This is to reiterate that they don't like what they're experiencing and would like to 'defeat' this.

> **Rosie:** I call him Glob because I don't like him, and I want him out of my life for good. When I listen to Glob, it makes me feel upset and angry. I feel happier when I don't listen to him.
> **Adult:** So Rosie, how does Glob make you feel?
> **Rosie:** I can't stand Glob. He is horrible. He is nasty. I hate Glob.
> **Adult:** How does Glob make you feel?
> **Rosie:** Glob makes me feel worried and anxious and sick.
> **Adult:** Why does Glob make you feel like that, Rosie?
> **Rosie:** Because Glob tells me to do things that I don't want to do.
> **Adult:** What is it that Glob tells you to do?
> **Rosie:** Glob tells me that I have to count things in multiples of two, otherwise something bad will happen.
> **Adult:** What do you say to Glob?
> **Rosie:** I tell Glob to shut up and go away.

Helping your child to fight Glob will help your child understand that they can win against these thoughts and behaviours. If your child feels that their behaviours are just something they do, then it is difficult for them to separate the disorder from themselves.

References and further reading

Allsopp, M. and Verduyn, C. (1989) 'A follow-up of adolescents with obsessive-compulsive disorder', *The British Journal of Psychiatry*, 154(6), pp.829–834.

March, J.S. and Mulle, K. (1998) *OCD in Children and Adolescents: A Cognitive-Behavioral Treatment Manual*. New York: Guilford Press.

The UK's Largest OCD Charity | OCD Action (2020). [Online] Available at: <http://www.ocdaction.org.uk/> (accessed 17 October 2020).

Salkovskis, P.M. (1999) 'Understanding and treating obsessive compulsive disorder', *Behaviour Research and Therapy, 37*, pp.S29–S52.

Veale, D. and Neziroglu, F. (2010) *Body Dysmorphic Disorder*. Chichester: Wiley-Blackwell.

Waite, P. and Williams, T. (2009) *Obsessive Compulsive Disorder*. London: Routledge.

10

Anxieties about health

Scott Lunn, Social Worker, CBT Therapist, & EMDR Therapist

This chapter explores children's anxieties about their health. Health anxieties are common in young people and can range from tummy aches to fear of brain tumours. The chapter provides an historical and cultural explanation for this particular form of anxiety, and looks into the different behaviours and thinking traps frequently experienced by children who worry about their health. The latter half of the chapter looks at some useful strategies families can use and metaphors that can help the child look at things from a different perspective. The aim is to develop your child's trust by working together and identifying possible behavioural experiments that develop alternative explanations for their focus about their health. As with any anxiety disorder, the concepts and interventions discussed must be considered in line with any professional advice sought should your child's anxiety become problematic and begin to seriously impact on their day–to-day functioning.

Andrew

Andrew is a ten-year-old boy who gets headaches, tummy aches and pains in his side and chest, and keeps going to his mum asking her if there is something seriously wrong with him. Andrew frequently worries that he has a serious illness and worries that he might die. His parents have taken him to see the GP and Andrew has been for numerous tests but they couldn't find anything out of the ordinary to confirm Andrew's complaints. Andrew often says, 'I don't think they looked in the right place or carried out the right test.'

Andrew's grandma died of cancer when he was nine. Soon after this he started complaining about his health; he is sure that illness runs in the family, and therefore that he is going to get cancer. Andrew spends a lot of time on the internet searching websites for known health conditions. His older sister refers to Andrew as a hypochondriac; Andrew's response is, 'but I have all the symptoms, therefore it must be true?'

There are a few possible explanations for Andrew's behaviour. Somatic – physical – symptoms or complaints are linked to psychological distresses and causes. Studies collated by Rutter et al. (2006) suggest that there is a high incidence of somatic complaints (physical symptoms) in children, particularly abdominal pains.

Health anxiety

Health anxiety (sometimes called hypochondria) is a condition that drives people to spend so much time worrying they're ill, or they might get ill, that it starts to take over their life. Those affected by health anxiety have an obsessional preoccupation with the idea that they are currently (or will be) experiencing a physical illness. The most common health anxieties tend to centre on conditions such as cancer, HIV, AIDs, and so on. However, the person experiencing health anxiety may fixate on any type of illness. Preoccupation with bodily symptoms and fear of suffering from a serious disease falls on a continuum ranging from a very mild concern about some unusual bodily sensation or observation to severe preoccupation and fear or conviction in individuals in whom thoughts and actions are centred around the overestimated risk of having or developing a serious, life-threatening illness (Salkovski et al., 1986).

Anxieties around health in the family

Neither health anxiety nor somatic symptoms are likely to just occur overnight, and often they are related to other factors in the child's life. It is important to consider the wider context of the behaviour.

It is helpful to think of behaviour as a form of communication rather than manipulation. For example, some behaviours associated with health anxiety may be to exert control; an example may be presenting with a severe headache and the child saying they can't go to school. Whilst this may be seen as the child making an excuse to not go to school, the underlying communication may be that they are feeling unsafe, they are struggling in a particular class, or they don't want to leave home as the child may be worried about their parent. Sometimes we need to look at the underlying communication and what it is related to. This could include the way the family functions together or difficulties in other areas of the child's life. This can be very difficult from within and often requires some external perspectives (and the very difficult task of sometimes being able to hear them!). We do need to be mindful that the child is one part of a wider system including the family, school, friends and community.

However, once a pattern has developed, it is often very difficult for the child to rationalize any other response. So, what can you do? In the example above, Andrew's knowledge about health conditions is so detailed that he can be very convincing, and what parent (or GP for that matter) wouldn't want to check it out just in case? Of course, you may have to do this in the first instance, and often NHS 111 will support that decision. However, as we point out later, if you're checking something out, you are assuming there is something wrong in the first place... Does this sound familiar?

Living with someone who has a preoccupation about their health can be very difficult, and it can be stressful when you are focused on your child's educational attainment and attendance. This health focus in the family can become intense and often exhausting, as the parent and child try and work through logical explanations, reassuring conversations and conflict between challenging the illogical and irrational thoughts, behaviours and seeing the child's distress heightening.

Not long ago, the term 'hypochondria' was used as a diagnostic term for health anxiety, however culturally, we have become a little impatient with people who are preoccupied about their health and the term 'hypochondriac' is largely used now in a derogatory sense. Psychiatric diagnostic manuals now refer to the term 'illness anxiety' and tend to only use the term *hypochondriasis* for more severe cases.

The Latin term *hypochondria* means 'abdomen' and later becomes linked with a further meaning which includes 'based on no real cause'. Over time this has created a negative connotation with the word, which we have all heard used jokingly. However, it is really important that we start by approaching this from a position of compassion.

To believe that you have something morbidly wrong with you, regardless of whether you do or not, is not very nice. So, starting from this compassionate position we are going to explore what constitutes illness or health anxiety:

- Preoccupation with having, or getting, a serious medical condition.
- Worrying that different body sensations are symptoms of a serious illness.
- On red alert to pick up concerns about your health condition.
- No reassurance from negative test results.
- Repeatedly checking the body for signs of illness.
- Avoiding people or places for fear of getting an infection.
- Constant talk about the disease and booking appointments with doctors or other professionals for reassurance.

People who are healthy can develop health anxiety, as can people who have a diagnosed medical condition. To qualify for a diagnosis of health anxiety disorder your symptoms must have persisted for at least six months and must have caused you significant distress, or adversely affected your daily life (American Psychiatric Association, 2013).

Helping your child make sense of what is happening

Primarily there are six areas that should be explored when someone is worried about their health all the time. These are:

1 Their beliefs about what is happening to them.
2 How avoidance or stopping doing things – for fear of making things worse can be unhelpful.
3 To review the level of checking – or constant body scans that are being undertaken to identify where there may be a problem.
4 To consider selective attention when focusing on that part of the body which will be amplifying the symptoms and feelings.
5 Looking at what reassurance seeking is happening, such as short-lived satisfaction from constant reassurance seeking from parents, health professionals, doctors, GPs, and so on.

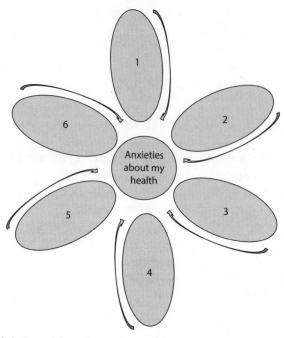

Figure 10.1 A problem flower for understanding health anxiety

6 Evaluating what information seeking is occurring, such as checking online to see what the symptoms might mean and for possible cures or treatments, this included the prognosis and percentage rates for improvement.

A useful way of pulling this together is to create a problem flower (see Figure 10.1). Take a blank piece of paper and draw a circle in the middle with six petals around it. Put your child's feared health condition in the middle and then think about the six themes above and start to consider these as petals to the flower head and each one reinforces the central belief.

Drawing this out can really help your child to visualize what is happening and to offer an alternative to the pre-existing belief that there is something physically wrong. This can be a very difficult transition, and in Andrew's case there is a fear that no one is taking him seriously. For Andrew, his parents need to validate his experience of worrying about his health and consider offering two different explanations for what is happening. By using a technique called Theory 'A' and Theory 'B', this considers the possibility of Andrew's symptoms to be explained from two different theories.

Theory A and Theory B

Let's consider that Theory A is Andrew's beliefs that something is wrong, that all the symptoms he's experiencing are real, and that this suggests they are related to a serious illness. Now, let's begin to estimate how much time through the week he is devoting to this theory (if we consider a week to be 168 hours). An example may be that Andrew is spending 60 hours per week devoted to his theory.

We now propose an alternative theory, Theory B. Theory B is that Andrew's symptoms could be explained through a psychological model and all of the behaviours that are identified in the flower drawn above, are what is maintaining Andrew's difficulties. We would then think with Andrew about what we might need to know to consider this theory and how we might start to shift some of Andrew's time to devoting to Theory B and to see if we could change or reduce some of the identified behaviours in the flower. By Andrew contemplating that there could be another reason for his difficulties, opens Andrew up to the possibility of change, which is what we are trying to achieve. (This approach is a well-known CBT technique that helps provide a framework from which to consider alternatives).

Taking the steps towards Theory A *and* Theory B, we might need some hard evidence of facts associated with the belief that Andrew has cancer. Actual numbers, pre-conditions of children with cancer, prevalence rates and associated complaints, and so on.

To offer a visual representation of Theory B, You could draw a picture of the body and identify how anxiety and worry affects how we feel physically, and where we might experience it in our bodies, see Chapter 1).

Try drawing the body and mapping out where and what the child is experiencing (see some examples below).

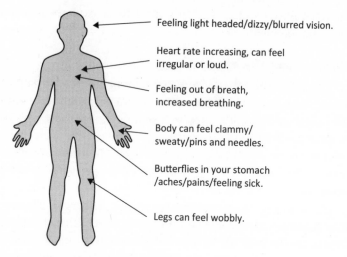

Figure 10.2 Body mapping example

The X-ray scan

A core behaviour of health anxiety is the scanning of the body and then the biased interpretation of the sensation or physical niggles that will follow this. By using the strategy of an X-ray scan, this can help offer support for Theory B about concentrating on specific parts of the body. Imagine with your child that they are in an X-ray scan: they are scanning their body from head to foot to find an area of the body that isn't hurting or not part of their health anxiety complaint (this may be the ankles and feet) and focus your attention on this area. Most people report experiencing an ache, numbness, a mild pain, pins and needles, and so on. All quite normal, but what does this highlight? In continuing to offer support for Theory B, it shows that if you concentrate on one part of your body long enough, that you will feel some physical sensation in it. This could help support Theory B, in that it is a psychologically driven sensation rather than a physical one.

By focusing our attention in one area we are, by default, looking for something. The body and mind can create feelings and sensations that are common to us all.

You are trying to link the scanning that is part of the associated behaviour of health anxiety with the question. You are asking if by scanning is it possible that we might increase the physical sensations and that, once we have identified them, we might then interpret these sensations as an anxiety and a threat to our health. This process of scanning, interpreting, further scanning and further interpreting can become a vicious cycle, resulting in increasing catastrophic thinking

An example of this increasing catastrophic thinking can be viewed in the figure 10.3. The earlier in the process you can stop the thinking the less distressing the thoughts will be.

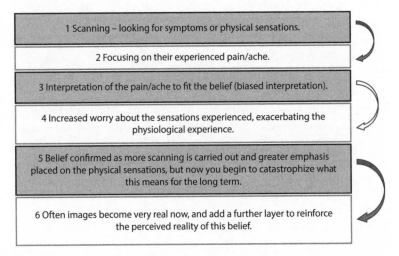

Figure 10.3

At stages one or two, it is really helpful to spend some time with your child measuring the level of distress or pain your child is feeling. This can be done on a 0–10 scale, with 0 being no distress or pain at all and 10 being the worst distress or pain it could ever be, or if it is a younger child, a horizontal line with a happy face at one end of the line and a sad face on the other, your child can then place a vertical line, through the horizontal one indicating how happy or sad they are feeling about their distress. Then between the stages indicated in Figure 10.3, do something that distracts your child from thinking about the X-ray scan for 20 or 30 minutes, make tea, play a game, go for a walk. When the time is up, rate that level of distress or pain. If the level of distress comes down, then this can support Theory B, in that if it was a physical illness such as a brain tumour or cancer, the level of distress or pain would be unlikely to reduce.

You are now getting closer to consolidating Theory B as an alternative perspective, but your child is still struggling to absorb and process this.

This next part of the journey is often the hardest, because we are going to ask your child to take a leap of faith. Remember you are asking them to go against all their pre-wired survival and evolutionary instincts, triggered by their belief that they have, or are at risk of, a serious illness (see Chapter 1). This is commonly referred to as the 'threat system' (the evolutionary system triggered by our amygdala which sends our bodies into overdrive in the hope of keeping the body/self alive) (Gilbert, 2008). Taking this next step is really difficult. We have to create enough curiosity and trust for them to consider that there may be an alternative – research suggests that using metaphors in practice, particularly with children and young people, can help them to find similarities, and can enable us to find a common language.

Using metaphors: a leap of faith

Using metaphors with children can be a great way of children learning to problem solve and subsequently help them to manage their own difficulties. The 'leap of faith' metaphor is used to try to help your child problem solve by using a story. You start by describing the situation below:

> Let's imagine you are going on a journey through a mysterious forest. You stumble across a village, and at the bottom of the village is a great temple. As you walk down towards the temple you come across the leader of the village, who is standing anxiously ready to

sacrifice one of the few animals left in the village. The village leader is responsible for all the villagers, who are dependent on nature, the land and its crops. The leader is surrounded by a group of villagers. The villagers are looking apprehensive. You ask one of the villagers what is happening. You are told that it's obvious – the village leader sacrifices an animal every day to make sure that the sun will rise in the morning. Without the sacrifice, the villagers believe the sun won't rise. This is because, every time a sacrifice has been made, the sun has always risen.

Ask your child how they might respond to the villager. You are aiming for your child to reach the conclusion that the sun will continue to rise without the sacrifice. You now continue with the story and the discussion between your child and the villager:

'The village is running out of food as nearly all the animals have been slaughtered,' the villager says, 'but at least we know for certain that the sun will rise.' The villagers are worried about how they might feed their families and they are worried that they may have to leave the village to find food elsewhere.

In getting your child to think what they might say to the leader and the villagers, take on the role of the leader yourself. Have your child and you, as the leader, problem solve the situation. Argue that you have always done it this way, and the sun has always risen. Your child needs to try and find a way of convincing you, as the leader, to consider an alternative belief. This is akin to using the Theory A/Theory B strategy. The village leader holds one theory (Theory A) and your child holds another theory (Theory B). Can your child create an experiment to test out Theory B? What can your child say to help the leader? What would it take for the leader to be convinced to take that 'leap of faith' and see whether the sun will rise without the need to slaughter an animal? What argument could your child offer to the leader to help them with their problem?

Once your child has helped find a solution for the village, you can use this metaphor to find similarities to their own situation. What can they take away from this and apply to their own difficulties?

In using this exercise to apply any learning to your own situation and keeping the Theory A and Theory B in mind, you begin to explore with your child how you might test an alternative theory to their belief that Theory A is the only possible explanation for their difficulties.

Identity – how illness can define who we are, and how we want others to see us

Sometimes there is a risk that your child can only really see themselves with their perceived illness. Perhaps they fear the alternative because of what it may mean to them without the illness. Sometimes this can be related to a fear of growing up, having more responsibility. Perhaps it is due to the related (secondary) functions of having an illness, which can include increased attention from you or other carers, school and health professionals. These can be seen as gains, even if they are negative responses. The perceived illness can sometimes define the child, so rather than them saying, 'I am Andrew', they may say 'I am Andrew and I have cancer'. On occasions it may be that they, and everyone else, have invested so much time into Theory A there is a reluctance to acknowledge Theory B due to worries about what others might say. This feeds into core emotions like shame and guilt. Also, there are routines developed, certain patterns of behaviour that can become the norm which also define the child around the illness. A useful question in these situations can be, 'What does being well look like?'. Some useful tools to visualize this include things like collages, collections of pictures, phrases, images, cartoons and the dreams that make you, you! You can do this on paper, or collect them in a folder on the computer or on your phone. This can help your child to develop a model of themselves when they consider Theory B.

Once your child has this picture of themselves, you need to start trying to map out how this person might begin to respond to health worries. The next step is then to start practicing these responses – always measuring what the perceived outcome might be, and what the actual outcome was. Your child, or you, should keep the outcomes in a journal. (A journal/notebook is really helpful to capture the work you have done, key 'light bulb' moments, reference to any learning, meanings or and tasks completed).

STOPP

Consider how they might start to re-interpret the physical sensations. A useful technique is using something called STOPP (getselfhelp.co.uk). This is a series of questions that help you to stop when you recognize a negative thought associated with a physical sensation or feeling. You are asked to consider if the way you are thinking about it is helpful? Is there an alternative way to think about the sensation or feeling? Can you take a look at what you are thinking and feeling right now from above and see it in context? This is very helpful to take your attention away from this moment right now and look at it over a longer period of time. There are some really helpful tools that you can use on the website above, particularly the STOPP process.

Summary

There are a number of useful tips and suggestions in this chapter which can be used with other anxieties and difficulties your child may be experiencing. The important thing is to help them develop a sense of trust that there is often more than one way to look at something. The way in which we look at a situation will change the way we feel about it, and behave. Remember you and the child's siblings and peers are the role models in this and they are trying to pick up subtle signals all the time to reinforce their beliefs. There is a helpful equation in chapter 11 that illustrates how we can have an overestimation of threat versus underestimation of coping. Working together to find the right balance between estimating the threat and how much your child can cope with, can be an effective strategy to use.

References and further reading

American Psychiatric Association (2013) *Diagnostic and Statistical Manual of Mental Disorders (5th Edition): DSM-V* Washington, DC: American Psychiatric Association.

Gilbert, P. (2010) 'An introduction to compassion focused therapy in cognitive behaviour therapy', *International Journal of Cognitive Therapy*.

Rutter, M. and Taylor, E. (2006) *Child and Adolescent Psychiatry* (4th edition). Oxford: Blackwell.

Salkovskis, P.M. and Warwick, H.M. (1986) 'Morbid preoccupations, health anxiety and reassurance: a cognitive-behavioral approach to hypochondriasis', *Behav Res Ther*, 24, pp.597–602.

World Health Organization (2018) *International Classification of Diseases for Mortality and Morbidity Statistics* (11th Revision). Available at: <icd. who.int/browse11/l-m/en>

Online resources

Anxiety UK: <www.anxietyuk.org.uk/anxiety-type/health-anxiety>
NHS, Health Anxiety: <www.nhs.uk/conditions/health-anxiety>
Getselfhelp:

11

Worries and panic

Scott Lunn, Social Worker, CBT Therapist, &
EMDR Therapist
Ann Cox, RMN & CBT Therapist

This chapter looks at worries about panic. Panic has a particular set of thoughts that makes it different from other worries and anxieties. This chapter will discuss these differences. We follow Abigail's difficulties throughout this chapter to help you understand how panic manifests itself and what you can do to help it. This chapter offers several strategies that you can do with your child to help overcome the symptoms.

Panic

Abigail

'I think I'm having a heart attack!'

Abigail is 14 years old and receives a notification from school that she needs to self-isolate for 14 days as she has come into contact with someone who tested positive for COVID-19. Abigail starts to breathe heavily and clutches her chest, she looks at her parents with a worried look and wonders what is happening. Abigail starts to cry: her parents provide some reassurance, telling her she's going to be okay and asking her to take some deep breaths, and try and calm down.

Throughout the period of isolation Abigail is very aware of her physical state and any potential COVID-19 related symptoms. On one occasion she begins to think about what might happen if she did get it. The physical feelings begin to intensify, she starts to breathe quicker, her hands feel clammy, her heart is beating faster and she again holds her chest and this time assumes she is having a heart attack. Abigail sits down for fear of falling over. Abigail's parents are concerned as this is the second time they have seen this happen; they decide to get her checked out by a health professional who suggests Abigail may have experienced a panic attack.

So, let's start at the beginning

I'm having a panic attack... Or are you? Let's look at what 'panic' actually means. A quick internet search pulls out the following phrases (Dictionary.com, 2020):

Panic
Noun:
- sudden uncontrollable fear or anxiety, often causing wildly unthinking behaviour
- sudden overwhelming fear, with or without cause, that produces hysterical or irrational behaviour, and that often spreads quickly through a group of persons or animals
- an instance, outbreak or period of such fear.

Adjective:
- of the nature of, caused by, or indicating panic: *A wave of panic buying shook the stock market.*
- (of fear, terror, etc.) suddenly destroying the self-control and impelling to some frantic action.

In Latin, *panic* means 'terror'! Let's look at what could trigger such a feeling.

We are going to break this down into two parts. In the example above, Abigail's initial feelings were triggered by receiving a letter from school. The second time was when she started thinking about what might happen to her and her family if she did get COVID-19. These are rational triggers and completely justified; however, what they triggered was an increase in anxiety symptoms, which again would be quite normal. However, what Abigail did next is what defines her difficulties to be defined by panic, in that she interpreted these symptoms into something more catastrophic – for example, having a heart attack. Children and young people can sometimes misinterpret these feelings, believing that they have a brain tumour, or that they are going to faint or be sick.

The second trigger can be based on an irrational thought or image:

Abigail noticed her hands were feeling clammy and immediately associated this with the fearful image of herself having a heart attack the previous week. This triggers a physical onslaught of anxiety-related symptoms which Abigail misinterprets again as confirmation that she has a weak heart and is having a heart attack. Abigail immediately seeks help from her parents and sits down again to stop herself from falling.

A study in the attendance of children at accident and emergency departments in 2003 highlighted that 12 per cent of patients attending A&E met the diagnostic criteria for panic disorder. Nearly two-thirds of all those suffering panic disorder seek medical advice at some point.

So, do you ring an ambulance, or dial 111? This is such a difficult call at this point as we will all want to err on the side of caution just to rule out that 'what if?', situation. I know, I've done it myself. But this is a learning curve and the very fact you are reading this book shows that you are already thinking that there might be something you can do.

Here's a very simple equation, which I have used in my clinical practice for many years:

$$\text{Anxiety} = \frac{\text{Overestimation of threat} \quad \rightarrow \quad \text{(misinterpretation of physical symptoms/catastrophizing)}}{\text{Underestimation of coping} \quad \leftarrow \quad \text{(reassurance seeking safety behaviours)}}$$

This equation has been referenced by leading cognitive behavioural therapists, authors, academics and therapists such as Padesky (2020) in the understanding of anxiety disorders. If you can imagine that the further the arrows move apart, the greater the feeling of anxiety. This is maintained by the top line (overestimation of threat), which is the way we think and behave in response to the situation or image. In Abigail's case, there is an apprehension that these physical feelings must mean something bad is going to happen. The threat mode is being switched on. This is reinforced by the bottom line (underestimation of coping) which is Abigail's belief, her learnt behaviour that she can't manage these symptoms because they are related to something out of her control. She starts to avoid situations and develops short-term strategies (safety behaviours).

The great thing about using this equation, and the diagram shown in Figure 11.1, is that you can use it (pinning it on the fridge door or inside a cupboard door, for example – somewhere

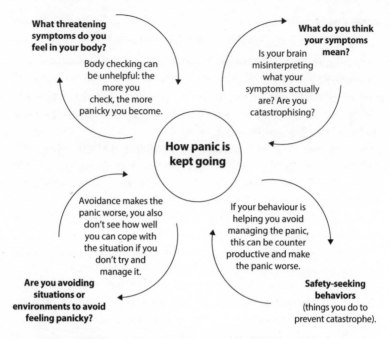

Figure 11.1 Diagram of what prevents panic from getting better

to hand) to begin to break down what you are doing or saying. The diagram above shows the top two cycles, which relate to the overestimation of threat, and the bottom two, which reinforce the underestimation of coping.

Your goal is to work with your child together to turn these arrows around, which can be done by:

- Learning about anxiety and the physical effects of this.
- Learning that there may be other explanations.
- Learning that you can manage anxiety and that it does go away after a while, normally after about 40 minutes (see Chapter One).
- Learning that every time you use a temporary solution (might be reassurance/might be taking deep breaths), while this may be useful in the short term, it is not always so in the long term.
- Learning that the language you use affects the way you think.
- Learning through experience that you can cope with anxiety, therefore reducing the catastrophic thoughts.

Language

The way we communicate in the family is very important – not only in the way we establish our relationships and use appropriate interactions in the way we communicate with one another, but also in the language we use. We use language to help create meanings, to establish rules and the ways we like to do things. Language helps us develop our values and beliefs in our family. The language we use to describe things like anxiety, worry and how we manage it, is often tied up in the way we are around each other. Families develop scripts (ways of communicating and behaving). Think about this, and about your situation.

The language you use will impact on the way you interpret what is happening. Often people find themselves falling into thinking traps, or thinking errors. These are statements or words that reinforce a negative meaning. For example, 'something bad is going to happen' (catastrophic thinking), 'this always happens' (generalization) and 'I should have done this' (self-judgement). This is a clear thinking trap or error because something bad *doesn't* always happen and the responsibility *doesn't* always fall on one person.

Compassion

In Latin, we know panic means 'terror', so remember, the whole experience can be very frightening indeed. Going back to the definition of panic at the start of the chapter, if we are caught in a cycle of irrational thinking, our understanding of what is real and what is not real may be unclear. Do not underestimate how terrifying this can be...

The threat system

In terms of panic, your child has the belief that something bad is going to happen due to the misinterpretation of physical symptoms, and a belief that they can't cope or manage them. Their evolutionary self-protecting system (the fight-or-flight system, as described in Chapter 1), is sending signals all around their body in response to this perceived threat. Blood is pumping around their body faster, they are trying to increase their intake of oxygen by breathing faster, blood is being pulled away from some organs (stomach, intestines and so on) so it can be sent to their muscles where it might be needed if their body needs to run or fight. Their body is on the lookout for danger, and your child may start to experience pins and needles, and sweaty palms.

All these symptoms are normal, but sometimes when the blood is moved away from the stomach nausea might be experienced; if your child starts to breathe more quickly and hyperventilate, their body adversely absorbs more carbon dioxide into their blood, which again can cause feelings of nausea, dizziness and pins and needles. If they understand these symptoms as those they know that happen in fight or flight, as opposed to catastrophizing them as a heart attack or a loss of control, this can help stop the thinking traps and errors and create irrational thoughts about the cause of the symptoms.

Safety behaviours

Safety behaviours are discussed in Chapter 1 also. In Abigail's case, grabbing her chest, sitting down and being comforted are all safety behaviours. Sometimes these strategies are helpful, but if they are used at the expense of Abigail learning that she would be alright without using the safety behaviours, there is a risk of reinforcing the fear that something might bad might happen. Safety behaviours can prevent us from learning how to cope. Families can sometimes get caught up with the child's safety behaviours, as they may look upon you to help lessen their distress. There is a fine balance to be had here, which many of us have experienced, for example, with children who don't sleep! Sometimes we have to use a firm approach to establish a routine, and reinforce the child's belief that they can sleep without all the safety behaviours we can become entangled in. Panic can be approached with a similar strategy.

Similarities with other types of anxiety

Often the word 'panic' is used when someone is experiencing acute symptoms of anxiety. As all symptoms across all the anxiety disorders will present with many of the same symptoms at times, panic can be very similar to health anxiety, for instance, in a fear of having a brain tumour, a person could present with intense symptoms, and with specific vomiting phobia, where someone will have intense symptoms when they think they are going to be sick. In both situation, the fear is not panic, but the symptoms experienced present similarly to panic. Please don't worry about labelling your child with the 'right' disorder! In all these circumstances the principles remain the same: the way we can make sense of it is slightly different, but overall we are looking at 'exposure' as the core treatment element alongside reducing the safety behaviours. Restructuring your child's thoughts (to challenge negative cognitions, thinking traps and errors) and building a positive model of self-coping is equally important. This can be incredibly powerful, and for anyone to face their fears and challenge some of their beliefs takes a lot of courage.

Strategies for managing panic

There are many strategies for managing panic. Chapter 1 has provided you and your child with some background about what anxiety is. It describes the basics of graded exposure, which is used to treat all anxiety-related difficulties in some form. Understanding the 'up' (fight-or-flight/sympathetic) and 'down' (rest-and-digest/parasympathetic) nervous system, and how this is managed in our bodies, is essential for all anxiety difficulties.

Fainting can be a real fear in people who have panic attacks. We saw in Chapter 1 that the 'up' ('fight-or-flight'/sympathetic) nervous system increases blood pressure and, therefore, it is highly unlikely that anyone would faint from panic or any other form of anxiety (except blood phobia, as this works in a slightly different way). However, if your child hyperventilates, which is where the person is breathing very rapidly and not taking full breaths, this can reduce the amount of oxygen in the blood and your child can faint because of this.

Below we have identified some strategies that can be used in ways of managing in panic, but can also be used for all anxiety disorders. Completing these regularly and more than once a day will have a positive effect on your child's level of anxiety and help them (and you) relax more often and more easily. The more you do them, the more relaxed you will feel. These are strategies that you and your child can do together, helping you to improve the connection with each other, and offering you some positive parent-child time.

Mindfulness

Mindfulness is a practice that helps us be mindful in the present moment, the here and now. It sounds easy, but it can take some practice; for example, what are you thinking about right now? Capture that thought. That thought has just taken you away from the here and now. Being present in the moment can be quite a skill to acquire. Mindfulness aims to help your child focus on the here and now, rather than on the past or the future. Mindfulness has an increasing evidence base, which means that it is proved to work in helping children regulate their mood and emotions, and that it helps in building resilience (Iacona and Johnson, 2018). There are many free apps that you can use for mindfulness, or there are script examples that you can search for on the internet; some of these can be found in the resources section at the end of this chapter. We'll look at one here, which uses a sultana (you can use anything similar).

Mindfulness practice

Firstly, get yourself and you child in a quiet, comfortable space. Then together breathe slowly and deeply. (Some people find it best to close their eyes when they do this.) Get you and your child to place the sultana in your mouth. Take some time to focus on the texture, the taste and how soft it feels in your mouth, how it is balanced on your tongue, how it is weighted there. A stream of thoughts will flow through yours and your child's mind. While you can both acknowledge them, you can both let the thoughts pass without following them. You and your child need to re-focus on the sultana, centring your minds in the here and now and letting the thoughts pass by. Spend time focusing on how your breaths flows past the sultana, breathing in and out, keeping it rhythmic, breathing in and out. The next time your breaths flows in, follow the breath gently to your chests, focus on the breaths, how it makes your chest rise and fall. Keeping both your thoughts in the present, focusing on the breaths, on breathing in and breathing out. Feel the breath flow through the full length and depth of your lungs. Feel your lungs suck the breath in and push it out through your mouths or noses, breathing in and breathing out. Acknowledge any thoughts that come into your mind, but let them pass by. Focus on your breath, feel both your chests rising and falling, think about how this feels in the top of your chests, how your breaths come from the lungs and up through the mouth and past the sultana, sweet and textured. Breathe in and out. Feel how the sultana feels in your mouths, the texture, how it is nestled on your tongue. Keep breathing in and out, in and out.

Slowly and deeply breathing, start to feel the breaths drawing from yours and your child's chest, towards your mouths, then exhale. Slowly, start to open both your eyes, and recognize you are back in the room together, still feeling the rise and fall of your chests. Take in the room around you and then you can both focus on moving.

The tricky aspect of mindfulness is allowing the thoughts, those thoughts that are not in the here and now, to pass through your mind without giving them attention. Keeping focus on the here and now can be difficult as our minds are so easily distracted. But it is easy to practice – you can do mindfulness anywhere.

Meditation and progressive muscle relaxation

Relaxation and meditation are long-term strategies used everywhere. As humans, we are always looking at how we can balance our wellbeing against the stressors of daily life. Meditation is similar to mindfulness in that the person doing it is more aware of their own body and what is happening to it. The main differences between meditation and mindfulness is that meditation generally has its tradition rooted in religion and spirituality (Keating, 2017). Meditation can be used similarly to mindfulness, with both focusing on spiritual wellbeing.

Progressive muscle relaxation

Progressive muscle relaxation helps your child focus on different parts of the body in a progressive way, helping the body and muscles to relax. It is helpful to do this relaxation lying on the floor, although it is not essential, as it can be done sitting down too.

Your child should start with their toes and feet, scrunch their toes and their feet up as tight as they can, hold for ten seconds, then release. Next, they move to the ankles: get your child to point their toes up towards their head as far as they will go, feeling the strain on the top of the foot and the ankle. They hold for ten seconds and then release.

Get your child to move systematically up the muscle groups in the body. Next, they point the toes to the floor, feeling the pull on the back of the calves, hold for ten seconds, then release.

The next muscles are the top of the leg. Your child can either lift their leg straight off the floor, then, hanging the bottom half of the leg (from the knee) downwards, make an upside down 'V' shape with their legs, moving to squeeze in their bottom, then the stomach, then their hands, then stretching fingers out to make a fist.

With their arms your child can make a sideways 'V' shape, or hold their tensed arms straight down, clenching their fists and then rolling their arms inwards. Tighten the chest, squeezing or rolling it inwards with the shoulders, then pull the shoulders up toward the chin.

Finally, get them to squeeze or screw up all the muscles in their face. All squeezing and tension should be held for ten seconds and then released.

Should your child wish to extend this relaxation, they can progressively move back down their body, tightening the muscle groups systematically, until they return to their feet. Progressive muscle relaxation is something you can do anywhere: it can help you focus on yourself and focus less on distractions.

Strategies specifically for panic

Hyperventilation provocation test

As we know, in order to reduce anxiety, we can use graded exposure to face the fear and ultimately reduce it. In managing panic, graded exposure is done by trying to replicate some of the feelings that may occur in panic. A simple strategy to try is called the 'hyperventilation provocation test' (Meuret, et al., 2005). Which, in laymen's terms, means to make yourself hyperventilate. By doing this we can replicate the symptoms that happen in the fight-or-flight response. Purposely hyperventilating will cause many of the same symptoms that occur in fight-or-flight. Demonstrating that you can bring on similar symptoms to fight-or-flight shows that you can control this somewhat in your body. What also helps to demonstrate this is that you can replicate the 'down' ('rest-and-digest'/parasympathetic) nervous system, too. Showing your child that by controlling your breathing you decrease the symptoms can be an extremely helpful strategy in helping them understand how they can help their body become less anxious. Again, this is something you can do together. (Please ensure that you read the information in Chapter 1 first, so that you can recognize the symptoms of the fight-or-flight response, and your child's panic symptoms.)

Hyperventilation provocation

Make sure you are in an environment where there is nothing you can fall over on or in to. Please be aware that hyperventilating can make you feel faint, so please stop the strategy if you this is the case – sometimes having a chair just behind you can be useful for you to sit in, should you need to. You can stop the test at any point you wish, even after 20 seconds of doing this breathing test you and your child can start feeling the symptoms. It should be noted that in my 20 years of practice I have never had a young person or parent faint doing this! For best results, do this standing up; you will still get some symptoms sitting down, but they may not be as many or impactful.

Start to breathe hard in and out very quickly, you should do this for about two to three minutes, although I struggle after two minutes. Your hard breathing cycle should be approximately two breaths a second. It is really quick. Once you are breathing in and out rapidly, you will quickly start to feel symptoms; once you feel them, name them out loud. ('Dry mouth', 'tingling', 'dizziness', 'chest getting tight', 'shaky legs' may be among them, but everyone is different, so it is interesting to see what your own are.) When you have reached as far as you feel you can, stop hyperventilating. Breathe slower and deeper, then say out loud how your symptoms are changing for the better. Your symptoms will quickly reduce when you stop hyperventilating. This demonstrates that you are helping out the 'down' (rest and digest/parasympathetic) nervous system to activate by slowing down your breathing, and because of this your symptoms reduce quickly.

Mimicking other symptoms of panic

Other similar strategies that can mimic panic are running up and down the stairs really fast (Hackman, 2004). Feeling the symptoms this produces, then feeling how quickly the symptoms reduce, can be helpful and helps your child to understand that symptoms will reduce given a short space of time. Spinning around in a chair (a wheeled chair) (Hoffman, 1999) can offer a similar experience. You can be creative in how you mimic symptoms and test out how your body overcomes them. Please ensure the environment around your child is safe when they try these.

Using a thought record

A thought record is a systematic way for a child to consider their thoughts in relation to a situation. They can weigh up the evidence for and against the thought; the idea is to come up with a more rational thought after going through this process. In this thought record, above, we will look at Abigail's example.

	Feelings	Rate feelings out of 100%	Evidence for the thought	Evidence against the thought	Re-rate feelings after evidencing the thought	More rational thought
Abigail became really anxious and thought she was going to have a heart attack.	Anxiety Fear Scared Worried	70% 100% 80% 70%	1) My body felt terrible, I had lots of anxiety symptoms, it really felt like I was having a heart attack.	1) I'm fit and healthy. 2) It is unlikely a 14 year old would have a heart attack. 3) I have felt like this before, and I have not had a heart attack. 4) Anxiety symptoms can make you feel bad.	Anxiety 40% Fear 70% Scared 30% Worried 25%	When I get anxious, I can fall in to thinking traps. Anxiety tries to trick you and you shouldn't always believe it.

Figure 11.2 An example of a thought record

Using a thought record can be really helpful as it can help your child think more objectively about the situation. What is important is that in the evidence sections, you must only include fact, not opinion. On all occasions, the evidence against the thought should be a longer list. This helps give a visual representation too; it can be helpful to number the pieces of evidence you are using to further illustrate the differences. Once your child gets used to using a thought record, they can be done mentally; it's a really helpful tool that I use in everyday situations to try and get perspective on a problem.

Summary

This chapter on panic has considered several strategies to help reduce panic symptoms in general and also to target specific feelings of panic. Panic can be very scary to the child struggling with it, but – like all other anxiety difficulties – it is very treatable.

References and further reading

Beck, A. (1976) *Cognitive Therapy and Emotional Disorders*. New York: Meridian

Dictionary.com (2020) Definition of panic: <www.dictionary.com/browse/panic> (accessed 1 February 2021).

Hackman, A. (2004) 'Chapter 3: Panic and agoraphobia', In: Bennett-Levy, J. et al. (2004) (eds.) *The Oxford Guide to Behavioural Experiments in Cognitive Therapy*. Oxford: Oxford University Press.

Hoffman, S.G. (1999) 'The value of psychophysiological data for cognitive behavioral treatment of panic disorder', *Cognitive and Behavioral Practice*, 6(3), pp.244–248.

Iacona, J. and Johnson, S. (2018) 'Neurobiology of trauma and mindfulness for children', *Journal of Trauma nursing*, 25(3), pp.187–191.

Keating, N. (2017) 'How children describe the fruits of meditation', *Religions*, 8(12), p.261.

Meuret, A.E., Ritz, T., Wilhelm, F.H. and Roth, W.T. (2005) 'Voluntary hyperventilation in the treatment of panic disorder—functions of hyperventilation, their implications for breathing training, and recommendations for standardization', *Clinical Psychology Review*, 25, pp. 285–306.

WHO (2011) F41.0 Panic disorder [episodic paroxysmal anxiety]. [Online]. Available at <icd.who.int/browse10/2010/en#/F40-F48> (accessed: 25 June 2020).

Padesky, Christine (2020) *Understanding Anxiety and the Anxiety Equation (Padesky Clinical Tip) – Part I* Available at: <www.youtube.com/watch?app=desktop&v=jw0ivpUQ43U>

Psychology Tools. *Panic attacks and panic disorder* <www.psychologytools.com/self-help/panic-attacks-and-panic-disorder/>

Zane, R. et al. (2003) 'Panic disorder and emergency services utilization', *Academic Emergency Medicine*, 10(10): <www.aemj.org>

Resources

Online tools

Psychology Tools: Panic attacks and panic disorder <www.psychology-tools.com/self-help/panic-attacks-and-panic-disorder/>

Mindfulness

Headspace <www.headspace.com>

NHS recommended mental health apps <www.nhs.uk/apps-library/category/mental-health/>

Oxford Cognitive Therapy Centre Resources, Relaxation Scripts <www.octc.co.uk/wp-content/uploads/2016/07/Relaxation-scripts.pdf>

12

Helping your child when something bad happens

Lisa Dale, CBT Therapist & EMDR Therapist

When a traumatic event occurs, as parents you will not only be potentially experiencing your own distress, but you will also be supporting your child with their own difficulties. This can feel like an incredibly challenging time for everyone. Your support, reassurance and guidance can make your child feel safe and secure. This chapter will help you to identify what a traumatic event is, different ways your child may react to these upsetting events and some ideas on how to support your child, while looking after your own wellbeing.

What is a traumatic event?

There are very many different events that can happen in life, and sometimes these are terrible events, such as witnessing a terrorist attack or a natural disaster or experiencing or witnessing a crime. Sometimes one-off incidents, such as a bullying episode at school, can be experienced as traumatic (these are often referred to as 'single incident traumas'). There are also more sustained and prolonged traumas that children and young people may experience. These might include prolonged abuse (sexual and physical), neglect, witnessing prolonged domestic violence, life-threatening illness and prolonged bullying.

Traumatic events involve the young person's perception that there is a threat to their life or significant injury. It is important to note that not all children who experience trauma will go on to develop Post-Traumatic Stress Disorder (PTSD).

Understanding traumatic memories

When trying to understand traumatic memories, try to imagine the mind as a factory production line. A crucial role of the production line is to process events that happen, so they can become memories. Most events are small and can be processed easily, but when a trauma occurs the production line finds it too hard to process, it's simply too large. As this event hasn't been processed it remains in the mind (staying in our present memory), which can make it feel like a current problem, reminders then continue to keep the problem alive. This can mean your child experiences intrusive thoughts and images that can cause significant distress. Sometimes, as a result, your child may avoid places or situations for fear of it happening again, which also reinforces the lack of processing.

Understanding how trauma can affect children

Children and young people can experience trauma in various ways that are unique and individual to them. Some will have symptoms immediately after an event, some will not experience symptoms for a few months, and some won't experience them at all.

Sarah

Sarah was involved in the Manchester Arena Bombing in May 2017. She was at the concert with her mum and a friend. Sarah was still in the main hall when she heard the loud bang and the floor shake beneath her. She remembered hearing screams and noticing everyone starting to rush towards her. She lost sight of her mum for just a few seconds. Sarah was not physically injured in the event, but has had lots of intrusive thoughts and images and since then, is having trouble sleeping.

Prior to the event Sarah was a keen dancer, and would regularly perform in shows. She attended school and was a well-liked member of the school community. However, since the event she has struggled with large groups of people, and is fearful of leaving her mum. When she attended school she felt a sense of panic, her heart raced and she found it difficult to catch her breath. Sarah found her thoughts were overwhelming. She started to have flashbacks and would go over the event in her mind. She remembered a small girl in front of her at the event; she is forever in Sarah's thoughts, wondering what happened to her that night. She is reliving the event on a regular basis. After hearing a car backfire or a crisp packet pop at school she is reminded of the event, and as a result her senses are ignited and she believes she can smell the smoke from the bomb. She worries about going to sleep for fear she will dream about the traumatic event. She talks to her friend about this, but the friend is not experiencing the same symptoms.

Anxiety after a traumatic event

The most common reaction after a traumatic event can often be a feeling of anxiety. Feelings of worry can present themselves in various ways, including as physical symptoms: stomach pains, feeling hot, shaky, breathless, extra trips to the toilet or feeling lightheaded. The physical symptoms are caused by the body's stress response. When we experience a stress response, our body produces more cortisol and adrenaline. This is the body's way of preparing to react to a threat, which is referred to as the fight-or-flight response (see Chapter 1 for more about this).

Sarah recalls: 'I didn't notice my symptoms to start off with, it was weird, a few weeks later I started to experience pains in my stomach, my heart would race and I felt physically sick. I didn't dare leave the house as I thought I would be sick.'

Sleep

Sleep can also be affected by feelings of anxiety. Your child may struggle to sleep, as they are experiencing intrusive thoughts and images. You may find your sleep is disrupted, as they are woken up by nightmares and may struggle to get back to sleep.

Avoidance

Intrusive thoughts, images and physical sensations can naturally make your child feel that they want to avoid anything that is remotely connected to the trauma.

Your child may display a variety of avoidance behaviours including:

- Avoiding talking to you or friends about what happened, as they may feel embarrassed that there is 'something wrong with them'. Young people can often feel cut-off from friends around them, who they feel don't understand.

- Avoiding places that are reminders of the event.
- Avoiding TV shows or songs with possible triggers: for example, if a child has witnessed domestic violence they may get distressed at the sight of blood in a film.

Sarah's own story shows the cycle of avoidance: when Sarah goes to her dance class, she feels anxiety with a distress level of 9/10 (10 being the highest anxiety), so she avoids the dance class and her anxiety goes down (3/10). Although it might appear to reduce the worry in the short term, this can be problematic in the long term as Sarah's life becomes more restrictive and she starts to feel worse.

Reliving and flashbacks

Your child may experience vivid flashbacks (these can be partial or full images of the event), which can feel like the trauma is happening all over again. These can happen at any time of the day or night and can often be very distressing for your child. The senses are often activated by smells: but sounds, visual reminders, textures and taste can all trigger a reliving experience. This can lead to your child experiencing emotions that they felt during the trauma.

There may be certain places that can trigger a flashback, or it can happen at random. Sometimes the flashbacks can last for a few seconds, sometimes for several hours.

> *Victoria*
> Victoria was sexually abused by her grandfather when she was five years old; she is experiencing flashbacks when she smells tobacco and beer. Her mum has recently started a new relationship and Victoria becomes increasingly distressed when in the presence of her mum's new partner as he smokes, and occasionally drinks beer. She has started to experience nightmares, particularly after contact with the new partner.

Nightmares

Nightmares of the event can be very intense and make it hard to separate dreams from reality. This can have a huge impact on sleep and can affect separation from you at bedtimes.

Other signs to look out for

Some of these symptoms may seem obvious, some less so. For example, in Sarah's case, her most obvious worry was attending another concert, for fear the event would happen again. However, some less obvious symptoms may include avoiding seeing or speaking to her friend because of a fear of embarrassment.

These triggers can create a strong anxiety reaction, and have a big impact on day-to-day functioning.

Change in emotions and behaviour

You may notice changes in your child's mood and behaviours. This could present as feeling irritable and angry, more defiant, your child may appear sad and upset, or they appear detached from their emotions. You may notice your child losing interest in activities they once enjoyed. They may find concentrating difficult at school or they are isolating themselves.

It is important to note that some of these symptoms can often be interpreted as depression and, if not assessed properly, can lead to an incorrect diagnosis and treatment.

> 'One minute I wanted to be out with my friends, the next I couldn't cope and would find myself back in my bedroom crying. I found it difficult just to enjoy the 'normal' things I had been used to doing before.'

Trauma in teenagers can be similar to trauma in adults; however, trauma in younger children can be very different. Children may revert to playing with toys like they did when they were younger, possibly re-enacting the event through imaginative play.

Suppressing the trauma

This might include avoiding anything that reminds your child of the trauma. It is common not to be able to remember the detail of what happened, or only part of what happened. Some children can disassociate, where they feel physically numb and cut off from their emotions. They may find it difficult to express affection.

It is also not uncommon for young people and teenagers to use drugs or alcohol as a means of coping with, and suppressing, the trauma.

Self-harm and suicidal thoughts

It may be that your child starts to experience urges to harm themselves or has suicidal thoughts. If this is the case, seek support from your GP or school to make a suitable referral to a child mental health support team.

Post-Traumatic Stress Disorder (PTSD)

PTSD is a recognized form of trauma that is diagnosable as a mental health condition. There are clinical criteria that need to be met in order for your child to be accurately diagnosed. This will be part of an assessment within a Child and Adolescent Mental Health Service (CAMHS). The recommended treatment highlighted in the NICE guidelines for PTSD is Trauma Focused Cognitive Behavioural Therapy (see the NICE Guidelines link in resources). This therapy can help your child to make the link between how our thoughts can affect the way we feel, and ultimately what we do. The treatment will include an assessment, formulation of what keeps the problem going and education on PTSD (so that young people and families know PTSD is a normal reaction to trauma). Supporting young people to talk, or write about, the trauma in detail, so that they can understand what has happened and update their memory, and helping young people encounter reminders of the trauma in a controlled way, so that their life becomes less restricted, is an important part of this treatment.

Eye Movement Desensitization and Reprocessing (EMDR)

EMDR is also recommended in the NICE Guidelines. EMDR involves an assessment to understand the trauma, providing education about trauma and how it is processed and a series of strategies to help manage the symptoms of trauma. EMDR involves making bilateral or two-sided movements, essentially this is left then right, left then right, whilst your child will recall the traumatic event. The bilateral movements (left, right, left, right) are intended to create a similar effect to the way your brain processes memories and experiences while you're sleeping. When you are asleep, you experience a process called rapid eye movement (REM) sleep, where the eyes move rapidly from side to side whilst you are asleep; which is said to process all of the day's events. When there is a trauma, REM sleep doesn't always process the trauma because it is too emotionally charged for REM sleep to do this. EMDR attempts to process trauma in the similar way to the REM sleep, but whilst you are awake, through the use of bilateral stimulation (left right, left right). For young children the processing of the trauma is often done through storytelling about the trauma, or through play, while the caregiver uses bilateral movements, for example, tapping on the child's shoulders (Shapiro, 2020). Both EMDR and CBT are recommended as having the evidence base to treat PTSD. Evidence-based therapy is any therapy that has been shown to be the most effective in scientific reviews.

Now that we have discussed different types of trauma and what to look out for, we can now look at some helpful strategies to consider supporting your child while they are waiting for their CAMHS intervention.

Strategies for helping your child after a traumatic event

All children and young people cope in different ways when they experience a traumatic event; there is no right or wrong way for a child to behave. Some will want to spend more time with others, some will prefer to be solitary. It is important that your child knows it is okay, whatever emotion they are feeling. It is 'normal' to feel this way, whether this is guilt, anger, frustration or sadness.

Talking with your child

Your child may look to you for reassurance after the event. They may ask questions to try to understand what has happened. Try to stay calm, give your child the time, share your recollection of the event, be honest and encourage your child to ask questions.

Sometimes talking helps, sometimes it doesn't! Don't pressurize your child, as sometimes this can make things worse. Just make sure they know you are there to listen when they are ready.

When they do want to talk about the event do not worry about saying the wrong thing. Just let them know you are there for them and you care. They may feel they want to talk about it over and over again. This is part of processing the trauma and can help your child make sense of what has happened. Your child might want to understand why this happened, and sometimes there is no answer to the 'why' question. Do not be tempted to tell your child to not go over it in their head. Validate your child's emotions so your child feels heard, and not criticized, for feeling a certain way, avoiding words like, 'you don't need to worry about that' instead rephrasing this to, 'I can understand this must feel difficult for you'.

Helping your child to feel safe and using appropriate affection is really important – for example, if a hug or touch can be difficult for your child, then a reassuring thumbs up, smile or pat on the back can help to give a sense of security and safety.

Talk of future plans; this can help reduce the feeling among young people experiencing trauma that their future is limited.

Structure and routine

Children who have experienced any type of trauma will feel more safe and secure when they have structure and routine. Maintaining bedtime routines, attending school and consistent family mealtimes are all important ways to help with this.

Distraction is helpful for a child to give them a 'break' from the worry they may be feeling. Encouraging play and activities can foster a good sense of normality.

If your child has experienced trauma from a specific event then try to avoid television coverage of that event; television can sometimes sensationalize events that can re-traumatize children.

Grounding techniques

Calm breathing

Using grounding skills can be really helpful for you and your child. When we feel anxious, our breathing can be affected, often giving a feeling of being overwhelmed. You can encourage your child to use grounding techniques to help with this, by helping your child to breathe in for a count of four, and breathe out to a count of four. Some good examples of scripts for this can be found on the *get self help* website while specific apps can also help with audio scripts (see helpful resources at the end of this chapter).

Compassion box and safe place

Building a 'compassion box' can help to ground your child when they are having a flashback, or are feeling overwhelmed. The idea behind the strategy is to collect items that make your child feel safe and secure, and remind them of better times. This could include photographs of family members, pets, friends, favourite smells, 'grounding' objects (precious rocks/stones), positive coping statements, favourite books and music to name a few. It's okay to start small. Your child may have some items he/she can immediately use and other items can be added over time. Your child could keep the bag close to hand to help them when they are feeling distressed and overwhelmed.

If your child is having a flashback, it might help to remind them that this is a past memory and you could say something like: 'This is the past, it's a memory. I know it feels really upsetting but it is not happening right now. This happened in the past. You are here with me, you are safe.'

The key is to constantly remind them that the event is in the past. It can help to write down the flashbacks as thoughts using the past tense, in a diary; this can also help to spot patterns in what triggers your child and their early warning signs.

Your child may also benefit from creating a safe place in their mind. This is a visualization technique which can be real or imaginary. Ask your child to think of a place that makes them feel safe. It is helpful to draw this picture, or write details of it, using the senses to pull out the details. For example, if your child's safe place is a beach you would say, 'what can you see in your safe place?' so, 'I see the calm water, the blue sky, the birds and the trees around me'. 'What can you smell?' 'I can smell the salt from the sea and the sweet smell of candy floss'. 'What can you taste in your safe place?' 'My favourite drink'. 'What can you touch/feel in your safe place?' 'The softness of the sea bed underneath me or the sand on my toes', and finally, 'What can you hear?', 'the birds and the soft waves crashing against the beach'.

Five senses

Another good grounding technique is being 'mindful' of your five senses when feeling overwhelmed. For example, you could ask your child to draw around their hand. For each finger write one the five senses: what can I see? What can I hear? What can I taste? What can I smell? What can I touch? This then becomes a portable strategy that can be used anywhere.

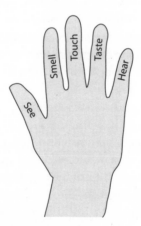

Figure 12.1 The five senses

Encourage your child to focus on noticing two to three things for each, to bring their attention back to the room and away from their worries, flashbacks or intrusive thoughts.

Whatever grounding technique you try, it's always best to try to practise these when your child is not feeling anxious. They are more likely to then use the strategies when they are feeling anxious. If you can set some time aside each day to practise these together and ask your child to rate their anxiety feeling before they use the grounding technique and then rate it after they have used the strategy, so for example, pre-breathing technique they may feel 6/10 anxious (10 being the highest anxiety) but afterwards they feel 2/10 anxious.

What school may be noticing

Schools can provide good structure and routine, mentioned previously in this chapter, however, in my experience the school may notice a change in your child's behaviour in the following ways:

- Struggling to concentrate in the classroom.
- Leaving the classroom due to anxiety
- Difficulties in relationships and friendship groups.
- Reduced attendance.
- Impulsive behaviour.
- Struggles with authority.
- Angry outbursts.
- Avoiding certain lessons.
- Reduced grades.
- Withdrawal.

If your child's school can understand that these behaviours are associated with trauma they are less likely to view the child's behaviour as disruptive and more likely to employ supportive strategies. These could include working alongside parents and mental health support services to develop suitable strategies that allow the child time out of the classroom to go to a safe place if needed, or having a direct link in the school your child can seek out when they need support. Schools can play an instrumental role in your child's recovery process.

Looking after yourself as a parent

In order to take care of your child in the best way, you need to take care of yourself. Share your worries with friends and family.

Look after yourself by trying to stick to a routine as much as you can. Exercise, eat healthy meals, and try to stick to a good sleep pattern. Without these, it can be much harder to manage the demands of parenting. Recovering from trauma can take time. If your child is about to start therapy, then be patient. Recovery is very much a journey.

Try to do further reading around trauma and PTSD, as the more you are aware of how this affects your child, the more you are prepared to support them and celebrate small wins – take note of the improvements your child has made.

Self-care is really important to keep you well, but also because of the potential for secondary trauma. This can happen from listening to the trauma. The more stressed and overwhelmed you feel, the greater the risk of secondary trauma. So, share your worries, try to keep to routines and use the grounding techniques discussed earlier in the chapter and take breaks where you can.

'You can't pour from an empty cup' – take care of yourself first! (Chapter 2 has more information on looking after yourself as a parent).

Where can I get support?

If you are concerned about your symptoms then you may wish to talk to your GP. Your GP can make the appropriate referral to counselling services and support, if needed.

Summary

It is important to highlight that the symptoms shown in this chapter are all typical reactions to an experience of trauma. This is a natural, human response to a difficult situation and with nurturing, understanding and treatment, (if needed); all members of the family can heal and thrive after the trauma.

There is life after trauma!

References and further reading

American Psychiatric Association (2013) *Diagnostic and Statistical Manual of Mental Disorders (5th Edition): DSM-V* Washington, DC: American Psychiatric Association.

Nice Guidelines: <www.nice.org.uk/guidance/ng116/evidence/evidence-review-a-psychological-psychosocial-and-other-nonpharmacological-interventions-for-the-prevention-of-ptsd-in-children-pdf-6602-621005>

EMDR Institute: Eye Movement Desensitizing and Reprocessing <emdr.com>

Online resources

For young people

YoungMinds Crisis Messengers: 24 hours a day, 7 days a week – crisis support across the UK. For urgent help you can text YM to 85258.

Samaritans: <www.Samaritans.org>

Childline: <www.childline.org.uk>

The Mix: <www.themix.org.uk>

For parents

YoungMinds parent helpline: 0808 802 5544

Child Mind Institute (2020) Helping Children Cope With Trauma (childmind.org)

EMDR Association UK, has some good resources and video clips on trauma: <emdrassociation.org.uk/a-unique-and-powerful-therapy/children-adolescents/>

Get Self Help: Trauma <www.getselfhelp.co.uk/ptsd.htm>

World Health Organization (2020) Doing What Matters in Times of Stress: An Illustrated Guide <www.who.int/publications/i/item/9789240003927>

13
Managing worries and physical health conditions

Dr Ruth Fishwick, Clinical Psychologist

Having a child who is unwell can be a stressful time for everyone in the family, whether this is a one-off, short-term (acute) illness or whether your child has a long-term physical health condition. Long-term conditions, sometimes called 'chronic diseases' are conditions for which there is currently no cure, and which are managed with drugs and other treatment. Hospital admissions, outpatient appointments and ongoing daily medications and treatments will be a feature of your child's 'patient journey'. This can throw up a number of anxieties for your child and for the family.

This chapter will focus on how to support your child if they have a long-term health condition, offering advice on how you can help your child throughout this journey. During this period you may experience emergency situations that do not allow time to prepare your child. Try not to worry; there are still helpful strategies that will work in these situations to reduce distress for you and your child and will be helpful should your child have a one-off 'acute' illness that requires hospital admission.

Think about a time when you or another family member may have been in hospital. What did you notice – what did you see, or hear? You may recall not understanding what was happening, not understanding the conversations that professionals were having in front of you, you may have memories of particular smells, or sounds. For children, 'the hospital is like a foreign country to whose customs, language and schedules they must learn to adapt' (Hall, 1987, cited in Rokach, 2016). And when children are scared, tired or in pain they become dependent on the safe and stable environment of their home, and the support of their family to be able to cope, feel strong and capable (Angström-Brännström et al., 2008, cited in Rokach 2016).

For children this is a vital necessity because their limited coping skills and emotional resources and resilience are not 'designed' to handle the tremendous amount of physical and emotional stress on them during a hospital admissions (Boyd and Hunsberger, 1998).

The journey through chronic illness

Pre-diagnosis

Your child might have been unwell for a time, and in order to get to a confirmed diagnosis they may need to have a number of different tests that are completely new to them (MRI/CT scans, X-rays, blood tests, scopes, etc). This may include having a general anaesthetic for the first time. They may be frightened about what is going on, and may seek support and reassurance that they are going to be okay, or will avoid discussions about what is going on. The best thing that you can do is to offer reassurance to your child by explaining that the medical team are doing the right thing by investigating, and that you will all have a greater understanding when the results are back. Avoid making promises to your child that you cannot guarantee that you can keep. For example, do not say that a procedure will not hurt, or that this is the last thing to be done, when it could be possible that more tests/procedures will be required. When promises are broken, children can start to lose trust in professionals and parents, which can have a negative impact on their relationships, and their patient journey.

While this is a stressful time for you all, it is important to recognize that your child will respond to your emotions. You are likely to be dealing with your own anxieties about the uncertainty of the situation, but it is important not to share your fears directly with your child. Share your fears with other adults but try to ensure that the 'adult' conversations do not happen in front of your child (or their siblings). This gives you the opportunity to talk with others about your thoughts and feelings without your children becoming worried about the child who is unwell, and their parent's fears.

At the point of diagnosis

Receiving a diagnosis of a chronic health condition for your child can bring a number of emotions: relief that you now know what is wrong and what you are dealing with; fear and uncertainty about what this diagnosis means because you do not know much, if anything, about the condition; and it can be a frightening experience for you and for your child. This journey is often referred to as a 'rollercoaster'. You may feel overwhelmed with the information, and your child may also experience this. Alternatively, your child may look like they have shut down, and may appear not to be communicating with the physical health team. This does not mean that they are not listening. Your child's healthcare team will try to make sure that your child has understood what they are talking about, in an age appropriate way.

Admissions to hospital

Medical teams aim to work with parents to keep children out of hospital as much as possible, and admissions will be managed for each child as an individual. For some specific conditions or for individual children there could be planned, routine admissions or there may be an increased chance that they will have more admissions to hospital throughout childhood due to the condition. Talking to your child about any planned admissions is important so that they know what to expect, and when. Think about important things coming up in the calendar that they would *like* to do (for example, a school trip) or something that they *need* to do (for example, exams). Let your medical team know, as they may be able to arrange the admission around this activity.

Outpatient appointments

Throughout the patient journey your child will have a number of appointments in Children's Outpatients, or Paediatric Outpatients as it may also be known. The main differences between an admission and an outpatient appointment are the location, and the length of stay. An outpatient appointment will be for a few hours. Outpatient appointments provide an opportunity to give your child a check-up with your physical health team, to start treatments like intravenous infusions, or to have brief procedures like blood tests or X-rays.

Strategies to support your child

There is no 'one-size fits all' approach here, but the strategies that follow are useful for hospital admissions and outpatient appointments.

Your child's support team

Help your child to think about who is in their support team. This can include particular members of staff from the hospital, teaching staff from school, close and wider family members, and their friends. If your child is struggling with an aspect of their care, ask them to think about what members of their support team might say to them.

Knowledge and understanding

You will have received a letter or phone call about the appointment. It is important to let your child know, reminding younger children right up to the day of the appointment. This will prevent difficult behaviours arising as a result of the shock and surprise of you and your child arriving at the hospital without warning.

If your team contact you to let you know that your child will need a procedure done (such as blood tests) then it is best to tell your child before this appointment to give them a chance to get used to the idea. This will give them time to think about the procedure and to tell you how it makes them think or feel so that you can share this with the team. If they are worried about what will happen, then the team and you can be prepared to support them using the strategies given in the section below, for example, the Hospital Passport, or by using technology or puzzle books as distraction.

Communication is key here. Trying to find the right balance is going to depend on the age of your child. If you share too much you may leave your child frightened or distressed. If you share nothing then they may also be frightened or distressed because they do not know what is going on, and what people (sometimes strangers) are going to 'do to them'.

Do you, as their parent understand what is going to happen at an appointment/admission? Spend time talking with your team to ensure that you understand about the situation, so that you and the team can find a way to talk to your child and so that you can support your child in between appointments. Find out what your child already knows and understands by asking them 'What do you think is happening/going to happen?' This can give an idea as to whether their knowledge is accurate or not, and whether there are any gaps that needs support from the medical team.

The more appointments you attend, the more you will understand what is expected of you and your child. It is important to talk about these experiences after appointments too. This will help to gain an understanding of how much your child knows and understands about what is being talked about.

Previous negative experiences can have an impact on your child, who may be firmer in their refusal to engage in a required procedure. Talking with your child, and supporting them to engage with their medical team offers your child the opportunity to share their fears. This gives the medical team a chance to make a difference, using the strategies outlined below and by giving your child a voice. Involving your child in developing their treatment plan guided by your specialist team allows them to feel more in control, in a situation where they often feel that they have none.

Infants and toddlers in particular may be frightened of having a physical examination during routine appointments. Ask your team if they can take pictures of all of the things that your child has to do throughout the appointment, and ask if you can have pictures of the team members. Your team, or you, can put together a picture book that you and your child can look at in between hospital appointments. They can also look at this independently, and this can increase the amount of exposure that they get to seeing themselves in a hospital environment.

With different treatments and medications, it is important to talk to them about what their medications are called and what they do, so that they become second nature and your child understands about how and why they need to take them. Your child's medical team will do this at different appointments.

Staying connected

Where possible it is important to support your child to keep in contact with their friends, family and school. Current digital technology enables us to have better communication and give children the chance to be connected with their peer and family support systems.

Relaxation

Teaching your child some simple deep breathing exercises, or relaxation exercises, can help to reduce anxiety in a stressful situation. You'll find some good examples of these throughout this book and they can all be very effective. In my experience, I have found it can be very helpful to support your child to imagine a 'safe place' (see Chapter 12). It is important that any relaxation exercises (including developing a safe place) are practised at a time when no other procedures are happening. It can then be practised throughout the admission and used for procedures with a good chance of success.

Having some home comforts can help your child to relax, for example taking their bedding and maybe their favourite toy. Other ideas include:

- Infants: playing peek-a-boo; having rattles; listening to lullabies; placing toys to encourage rolling, crawling, kicking.
- Toddlers: listening to music; stacking blocks; Play Doh; scribbling with crayons; watching TV.
- Preschool: drawing; reading with an adult; cutting and sticking; bouncing/throwing/catching balls.
- School age: reading; puzzles; arts and crafts; board games.
- Adolescent: playing card/board games; playing on computers/tablets/video consoles; listening to favourite music; watching films.

Children's wards have play specialists who will be available to provide tasks appropriate for your child's age and ability.

Physical contact

Rub your child's back/arm, stroke their forehead/cheek. Try not to be offended if they push you away, as some medications can leave them sensitive to touch – if your child does this, talk in a calm voice and ask them to put your hand where they think it will be helpful.

Naming emotions

Hospitalized children are often confused, frightened and in need of support, reassurance and an explanation of what they will be exposed to [in a manner that fits their level of maturity], and mostly, they need to be recognized as 'little people' who are keen to be treated not just as 'bodies' but as humans with emotions, pain, illness and concerns (Rokach, 2016). Feeling helpless, along with the fear and pain, can leave children feeling powerless. The aim of the hospital staff is to reduce the risk of trauma to a child and their family as a result of a hospital admission. Being confined to a bed, bay or side room can leave your child feeling like they are trapped or stuck no matter how long they are in hospital.

Due to their age and/or cognitive development children will express their emotions through behaviour rather than through words. Sometimes children need help to understand and express how they are feeling emotionally. Lots of emotions will be coming up for your child. For all children, but especially for the younger ones, it is important to name the emotion for them, for example: 'I think that the idea of having a blood test is making you feel worried and upset.' By naming the emotion, you are shaping your child's emotional vocabulary, and increasing the chance that they will be able to communicate the emotion in the future. You are also giving them a chance to tell you if you have got the emotion right, or wrong. You will need to do this across different situations (health and non-health related) to help them recognize when new emotions arise, and when the same emotion comes in different situations. You can also reflect with your child about times when they have been successful in overcoming difficult situations to help build their confidence.

Try to avoid using the word 'brave' – this word is brilliant to encourage your child when they have succeeded with a procedure. However, if your child is not able to go through with a procedure that previously they have felt 'brave' for achieving, they may begin to have feelings of doubt and think that they are a failure. Normalize the situation for your child, for example, 'it's okay to feel scared', then be curious with your child as to what might make the situation easier for them.

Hospital Passport

During an admission it is likely that your child will need to have procedures done that they have not experienced before (or they have experienced lots of times). Children of different ages may experience anxiety about procedures, and they may cry, scream, refuse verbally or refuse by using their arms/ legs to prevent the medical professional from having access to their body. A lot of this 'resistance' can be them trying to take back control in a situation where they feel they have none. They may find themselves in unfamiliar situations, and may see that resistance is the only way to regain control and delay, or even stop procedures from happening. Your child may then learn that this is an effective strategy to stop things from happening, and may repeat these behaviours, or increase them if necessary.

Hospital Passports currently come in a variety of forms; some can be several pages, and have pictures to support children with learning disabilities to feel involved and empowered. To help shift the idea that 'things are being done *to* them' to the idea that 'things are being done *with* them', Hospital Passports can be used with patients of different ages, working with all members of the physical health team to work out what can be possible.

Hospital Passports are very effective, particularly when the individual passport is tailored to the child for a specific situation. This can help them feel supported, and like they have some control over the situation. It also offers the opportunity to personalize the Hospital Passport with images of what the child's likes and dislikes. Hospital Passports encourage children to work with hospital staff rather than against them. They are also really useful if children find it difficult to communicate their fears with health professionals.

To create a Hospital Passport, talk to your named nurse on the ward or ask to speak with the play specialist team. There may also be a clinical psychologist in your specialist team who could do this piece of work. Figure 13.1 shows the simple structure of an effective Hospital Passport suitable for James in the following case study. It includes name, age, what the hospital staff need to know (for example, what the child is fearful of), and what staff can do to help.

James

James is a 14-year-old boy with cystic fibrosis who lives with his mum. He also has some autistic traits. As part of cystic fibrosis care he has to have regular long-line intravenous (IV) antibiotics and over time James' veins have become scarred from numerous long-line IV antibiotics, which made it difficult to complete full antibiotic courses.

When James was four years old, he had a port-a-cath inserted just underneath the skin in his chest. The port-a-cath is an implanted device with a self-sealing silicone bubble, and a plastic catheter. It was hoped that this would make IV antibiotics easier for James, and these were initially successful. After three years, the port-a-cath became difficult and painful to flush. A chest X-ray demonstrated that the catheter attached to the port-a-cath had become disconnected and migrated. The catheter was retrieved by the interventional radiology team using a multi-snare. James made a full recovery and a new catheter was fitted.

Over the next few years James started to develop anxiety immediately before each port-a-cath flush and required a 'safe hold' from his mum, his older brother or a member of staff to support him through the procedure. With increasing resistance from James, and his feeling of being out of control, the port-a-cath flushes became more dangerous for James and the nurse administering the flush, so the cystic fibrosis team asked me to work with him. James was too anxious to say what made it difficult, but on further exploration he recalled the moment the consultant showed him the catheter that had been retrieved. He was scared when he saw the catheter and linked the broken catheter to any future port-a-cath flushes. He became worried that every time the port-a-cath was accessed it could break, so would refuse and delay the flush procedure, which added to future anxiety. Giving James some control and decision-making helped him to overcome the difficulties having the port-a-cath accessed.

The port-a-cath became infected and required removing. This was more evidence for James that the device that had been supposed to make things easier for him, could go wrong. James was scared of the procedure, the general anaesthetic and waking with a long-line for a course of IV antibiotics. Above all else he was scared that a new port-a-cath would be inserted after a period of recovery. Having already had two problems with his port-a-cath James was convinced and worried that more things could go wrong.

My Hospital Passport

Name: James
Age: 14

My name is James and I am very nervous about having a general anaesthetic to remove my port-a-cath. I do not like the feeling of having a general anaesthetic and I will fight against it. I feel scared because of previous experiences of general anaesthetic and surgery. I am worried about being in pain after the operation.

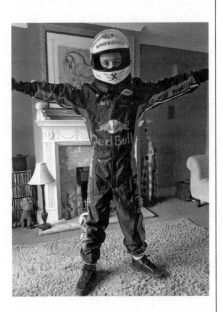

This is how you can help me:

- No sleepy pipe and mask.
- Please do not talk about what you are going to do in front of me.
- Please do not show me the port-a-cath afterwards.
- Please access my port-a-cath on the morning of my operation.
- I would like a Diazepam (tablet form) on Monday night and Tuesday morning and to relax watching F1 videos.
- I would like to clamp and unclamp my port-a-cath so you can push through the flush/medication.
- Please ask me to rate my pain out of ten.

Figure 13.1 A Hospital Passport for James

The Hospital Passport is kept with your child's health record, and your child will also be given a copy. Having personalized pictures can help healthcare professionals to get to know your child by providing a topic of conversation before getting to the health 'stuff'. The Hospital Passport can be useful for general aspects of an admission, or for specific aspects of care that provide more anxiety for your child.

Supporting your child at home

Children crave structure and routine to help them to feel safe and secure. A good bedtime routine can improve your child's sleep habits, for example, and adhering to family routines is important for family resilience in times of crisis (Black and Lobo, 2008). You can support your child to navigate the challenges of their physical health journey by making sure that you do not start to break your own rules: suddenly allowing them to stay up late; giving extra days off school; or less chores to do causes them to feel confused. Sticking to a daily family routine is important. Having set roles for each member of the family will help your family home to run smoothly. This will support you should an emergency admission catch you off-guard.

As your child grows up they will need to learn the activities of daily living appropriate for their age, for example, tidying their bedroom, setting the dinner table, washing, cooking, cleaning, and so on. It is important to factor these into their day alongside their daily medical requirements to help them to adjust to the demands. While there is little point expecting a child experiencing a flare up of asthma, or arthritis to tidy their bedroom, it is important at other times to ensure that they keep up with their responsibilities, and that you have a discussion about what is expected of them during good and bad days. This will help to create a healthy balance and will prepare them for the next stages in their growth and development.

Riding the difficult times

It can be difficult to manage the daily needs of a chronic health condition while balancing your child's need to grow socially and emotionally. At some point in your child's life they may start to rebel against the condition and its medications/treatments. This can raise your own anxieties, which in turn may impact upon how you respond to your child's refusal. It is important to remain calm and talk to them with a calm voice and explain the reasons for their treatment. Ask your child 'what makes it difficult to keep up with treatments?' Be curious with them, find out whether they understand the consequences of making a choice not to do treatments. Common reasons for wanting to stop treatments include:

- They may feel tired and bored of doing the same thing every day.
- They may have noticed differences between them and their friends, or that they feel they do not have the same opportunities.
- They may not understand the consequences of stopping treatment.
- They may express sadness or anxiety about falling behind at school.

Encourage them to share with you how they are feeling, so that you can discuss this with their teachers. Once you have an understanding you can talk with your medical team. It may be possible to review medications and treatments to reduce the burden.

Supporting your child at school

If your child has had a period of time out of school due to appointments, an admission or an operation, they may be worried about questions that people at school may ask on their return (about their absence, about medication such as insulin or enzymes taken at break or lunchtimes, or about visible medical devices such as a naso-gastric tube/PEG). You can help them by thinking about a script you can rehearse with your child for them to use in order to satisfy curiosity without giving too much away. It can help your child to think with you about how much they want other people to know, they may want to bring humour into the script.

Your child may be worried that they are going to fall behind their peers academically, or they may have found that they already are. This can bring an additional anxiety about education that you may not have recognized in your child before. Talk with your child's class teacher/head of year/pastoral leader/ special educational needs co-ordinator (SENCo) about any new diagnosis, or any changes to your child's treatment. Should your child require an admission, talk with your child's medical team about whether there is a Hospital Education Team available. The teachers there are able to liaise directly with your child's school to establish where your child is up to academically and will try to cover work during your child's admission.

Your self-care

As a parent, you may go into overdrive thinking that your role is to care for your child and make them well again. It is important not to neglect your own physical and emotional needs, and to engage in positive self-care. If you can bring down your own stress levels, then you child will benefit from this and their own stress levels may also reduce. Not all these strategies will be possible for everyone, but here are some that have proved helpful to parents I have worked with over the years:

- Having comfy clothes to wear while on the ward.
- Bringing your own duvet.
- Wearing an eye mask.
- Bringing an iPad/tablet/book/magazine.
- Taking time off the ward.
- Understanding how you feel about hospitals/procedures.

If you struggle with any aspects of your child's care, do not be afraid to ask for support. We need to look after you, as you are a big part of your child's support team (Chapter 2 offers more information about looking after yourself as a parent).

Take-away message

Your child will experience highs and lows along their physical health journey. Your team want to increase the number of highs and reduce the number of lows that happen in this time, and want to work with your child. Education is key throughout this journey so that your child can ask questions, and understand about what they are expected to do every day. There are a number of different strategies in this chapter and book that will be helpful, but if you find that your child continues to struggle with anxiety about procedures, admissions, their chronic health condition, or any combination of the three then it may be helpful for them to talk to your local Paediatric Psychology Service, who are Clinical Psychologists with experience of supporting children with chronic physical health problems. For further support, please consult *When Your Child is Sick: A Guide to Navigating the Emotional Challenges of Caring for a Child Who is Ill*, by Joanna Breyer (2021).

References and further reading

Black, K. and Lobo, M. (2008). A Conceptual Review of Family Resilience Factors. *Journal of Family Nursing* [online] 14(1), pp.33–55. Available at: <journals.sagepub.com/doi/abs/10.1177/1074840707312237> (accessed on 15th June 2020).

Boyd, J.R. and Hunsberger, M. (1998) 'Chronically ill children coping with repeated hospitalizations: their perceptions and suggested interventions', *Journal of Pediatric Nursing*, 13, pp.330–342.

Breyer, J. (2021) *When Your Child is Sick: A Guide to Navigating the Emotional Challenges of Caring for a Child Who is Ill*, London: Sheldon Press.

Rokach, A. (2016) 'Psychological, emotional and physical experiences of hospitalized children', *Clinical Case Reports and Reviews*, 2(4): pp.399–401 Available at: <www.oatext.com/Psychological-emotional-and-physical-experiences-of-hospitalized-children.php#gsc.tab=0> (accessed 15 June 2020).

14

Worries, self-harm and suicidal thoughts

Dr Laurence Baldwin, RMN

This chapter is a little different: it is about a symptom, but a symptom that can be very scary for the young people who experience thoughts about harming themselves, and very scary for the people around them too. The ways in which anxieties and worries (and other thoughts too) can show themselves can be very emotive, so it is important to think about the emotions that self-harm generates in all of us, as well as looking at ways to help young people who suffer urges to harm themselves, or even to try to end their lives.

Why is this chapter here?

On first glance this may seem to be a strange chapter to have in a book on overcoming anxieties, but self-harm is a very common symptom of people, especially young people, who are anxious. There are other reasons why young people, and even children, will hurt themselves, but anxiety is a very common one, which is why we are talking about it here. The most important thing to remember is that self-harm is just that, a symptom of something else. That something else may be anxieties or fears, it may be that something bad is happening to the child or young person and they can't find a way to talk about it to a trusted adult, or they don't feel good about themselves for some other reason. But self-harm is not a condition in its own right, it is always an indicator of something else going on. It may serve a function, an idea that we will look at in this chapter, but is not something that can be 'cured' in itself, without getting to the root of why the young person chooses (or feels compelled) to hurt themselves. It's also distressing for parents and people around, as well as for the young person themselves, so it's important to be able to recognize those feelings in ourselves as part of trying to be helpful.

'Some young people do it for attention, like I did when I first started. That doesn't mean they should be ignored. There are plenty of ways to go and get attention, why cause yourself pain? And if someone cries for help, bloody well give them it, don't just stand there and judge the way in which they're asking for it.'

Young person, quoted in 'Truth Hurts'

Definitions of self-harm and suicidality

The words we use around this subject are quite important, especially the words we use in front of, or in the earshot of, the young people who are involved. Words are important because they express what you are thinking about a subject, especially an emotive subject like self-harm, and they also can be loaded with the sort of judgements which young people are particularly sensitive to. Most of the literature on self-harm will no longer use the phrase 'deliberate self-harm' (DSH), for example, because this is seen as quite blaming. It's not a long step from 'deliberate self-harm' as a phrase, to 'you did this to yourself' and therefore 'you don't deserve my sympathy or understanding'. Of course, it is possible to justify this phrase as a way of differentiating this from 'accidental self-harm', but normally we can just call these incidents 'accidents' anyway. Given that one of the most important things to do in order to help children and young people who self-harm, is to try and establish trust, and a helping relationship, using language which is blaming or potentially stigmatizing will get in the way of that young person taking that first step of trusting in the people around them. Young people often report that the attitudes of staff in emergency departments, for example, are negative towards people who self-harm, as they are seen as self-inflicted wounds and somehow not worthy of the same level of compassion that is given to other patients who may just be seen as unfortunate enough to have been injured some other way. A lot of work has been done on destigmatizing self-harm, but the reported experiences of young people who attend emergency departments suggest that more work still needs to be done.

The difference between self-harm and suicidal behaviour is important to understand because they are very different, although there is a link. The most important element is about intent: what was the young person thinking would happen as a result of whatever they did? If they thought they would die (even if the method they used wouldn't actually have killed them) then that is 'suicidal intent' and needs to be taken as a serious safety (or risk) issue, and a safety plan (or risk assessment) put in place to prevent future potentially fatal incidents. Mental health staff have systems for assessing risk, and intent, and should put these systems in place, and may also need to involve Safeguarding Children staff from social work departments, or from the hospital's own safeguarding team. Safeguarding Children is the term that is now used in place of Child Protection, and is governed by a whole system which is mandatory for health and social care staff in the UK. An important factor in children and young people is that the intent is important even if the action wouldn't have ever killed them. If you have always been told, for example, that you should never take more than two paracetamol because taking more could kill you, then taking four paracetamol, thinking that it *will* kill you, is still suicidal intent. This may sound strange, but it is based on a real incident. Not knowing that it wouldn't work doesn't mean that the idea has changed, the intent was still there. Even if this intent is brief (technically 'fleeting intent') it needs to be subject to a thorough mental health assessment and safety planning. Just because it has passed for now doesn't mean the thoughts won't come back. So any suicidal intent, from fleeting thoughts, to more long-term planning, needs to be taken very seriously, with measures taken to ensure that both the short-term risks are addressed and a longer term plan put in place to deal with the underlying issues which are leading to these thoughts and actions. Talking about this issue is also difficult, but it is a myth that talking about people wanting, or not wanting, to kill themselves, will make them more likely to try it. There is a lot of research now that tells us that this is not the case, just asking won't give people the idea to try and kill themselves, but it will let them know you are very worried about them, and taking them seriously.

People who self-harm without intending to kill themselves, which is most people, should not be treated any less seriously. But it does mean that the underlying motivation is different. It means we still need to see the action of self-harming as having meaning, just that the meaning is not to try and end one's life. Research does suggest that people who self-harm are at greater risk of suicide in the long run, if the causes of the distress that leads to them self-harming are not addressed. As we noted earlier, self-harm is a symptom of something else that is distressing, and it is usually the only way that young people have of coping with this 'something else'. This was the most important finding of the Mental Health Foundation's national enquiry 'Truth Hurts'. It's a tough read, but has a lot of insight into the issues, based on talking to a lot of people, younger and older, who have self-harmed.

Self-harm comes in a lot of varieties, the most commonly seen ones are self-poisoning (overdosing on medications or illegal drugs), and cutting, either hidden or openly. There are, of course, a lot of other ways of harming yourself, but these are the most common in children and young people as medication, and the tools for cutting are easily available in the home, or bought at a shop (no one ever stopped a child from buying a pencil sharpener, but they do contain a sharp blade!). Self-harm definitions do not usually include other long-term, potentially damaging actions such as self-starving, use of illegal drugs, smoking or drinking excessively, or putting yourself in danger through reckless sexual activity or participating in dangerous sports. These would be seen either as symptoms of other problems (anorexia or eating problems), or even normal developmental acting-out or risk-taking. Some self-neglect of proper medication regimes, however, can be classed as self-harming, such as people living with Type 1 diabetes mis-managing their insulin with the intent of putting themselves into a diabetic coma. Again, this needs to be seen as a symptom of underlying distress.

There are some other social and developmental considerations to take into account when thinking about self-harm. We highlighted the intent behind the actions, and for some younger children they may refer to things that they don't fully understand. Very young children, for example, don't have a fully formed idea of the permanency of death, so a five-year-old saying that they want to kill themselves is very distressing for the adults around them to hear, but it is unlikely that they have the same intent as an older child or young person saying a similar thing, when they do not fully understand what they are saying. It still obviously needs to be taken as a symptom of underlying distress, however, and the child should be helped in a sympathetic way to cope with their emotions. We have a curious way of trying to soften the blow of family deaths for children, talking of people being 'at peace' or 'in a better place', but these can be easily misunderstood by them. If they desperately miss a grandparent who has recently passed away, they may want to be with them and express themselves as wanting to be in heaven with them, rather than here, as a way of coping with their sadness and bereavement. Socially, there are also things that need to be taken into account in trying to understand the actions of young people. Statistically, young women are more likely to self-harm (though this is also socially changing and many more young men are self-harming now) and men (including young men) are less likely to talk about their problems and resort to more violent means of self-harm when they cannot cope any longer. Some cultural pressures lead to higher rates of risk within Black and Minority Ethnic group young people, and we know that being a care leaver, or being LGBTQ+, places additional stresses on those groups of young people, meaning they are at greater risk.

> I was very confused about my emotions when I was young. It was considered to be attention seeking to cut yourself and I didn't want attention. I just couldn't control my emotions. I needed an outlet. I was ashamed of it. Which really just added to my problems as I already felt ashamed of other things in my life.
>
> Young person, quoted in 'Truth Hurts'

Why do they do it?

The idea that self-harm is a symptom of something else is borne out by research that has looked into the reasons behind self-harm incidents. Many areas in the UK now have dedicated liaison teams for children and young people who present with self-harm injuries at emergency departments, and there is generally an increase in admissions during the period leading up to exams in May and June each year. The pattern has changed recently, so that throughout the year there is a more consistent demand now. NHS services follow clinical guidelines issued by the National Institute for Health and Care Excellence (NICE), which has two sets of guidelines for self-harm (short- and long-term management). This usually involves an admission to a children's ward to allow an assessment by a mental health professional, following initial treatment of injuries. For some young people this may be to a Medical Assessment Unit (MAU) instead. This NICE guidance means more young people are being seen, as awareness in the community (among primary care staff, social care staff and teachers) of the importance of hospitalization is stressed, which may explain why the rates are more even across the year.

The top reasons given by young people as causes of their self-harm are:

- Being bullied at school.
- Not getting on with parents.
- Stress and worry about academic performance and not getting on with examinations.
- Parental divorce.
- Bereavement.
- Unwanted pregnancy.
- Problems to do with race, culture or religion.
- Low self-esteem.
- Feeling rejected.

Additionally, the stress involved in these two issues adds further high risk factors:

- Experience of abuse in earlier childhood (whether sexual, physical, neglect and/or emotional) – severe and prolonged sexual abuse is known to lead to a higher incidence of self-harm.
- LGBTQ (lesbian, gay, bisexual and transgender) young people are estimated to be two or three times more likely to self-harm

than heterosexual young people, and homophobic bullying at school is implicated in higher rates of self-harm.

All of these issues relate to anxieties and worries, and we can again see self-harm in the developmental context of young people growing up and learning to cope with things that they have not previously experienced. The incidence of self-harm admissions in the run up to exams is a good example of this. My own experience, while leading the young people's self-harm team in my own area, was that many young people actually did not directly say it was the exam stress that was the immediate cause of their self-harm episode, they usually talked about other things worrying them, but it was clear that they were coping with their first period of sustained anxiety, and their ability to cope with other issues was affected by this underlying worry. So young people learning to cope with exam anxiety, despite the support that schools are better able to offer now, find this new experience very difficult.

Likewise, as young people grow older, they are massively affected by the sense of how they are perceived by their friends and others around them. This stage of separating from parents and family as the main support, and being much more aware of what their friends think, and trying to find their own identity, is a normal phase of development. But not coping with things simply piles on the pressure and makes them think they have failed. Not fitting in, or being unusual in any way, becomes a pressure which is difficult to share. This pressure is particularly true for LGBTQ+ young people, who are likely to be subjected to a lot of bullying or abuse from their peers, which impacts on self-esteem. For many the sense of isolation which comes from being 'different', either for being lesbian, gay, bisexual, trans or queer, or indeed from having a disability, or being neurodivergent (as we discussed in Chapter 6), means that anxiety levels skyrocket, and self-harm may be one of the ways of coping. Even in the digital age, finding others like yourself, and learning better coping mechanisms, or seeking support, can be very difficult, even once the stage of recognizing which group you may actually belong to has been achieved.

Young people will self-harm for a number of reasons. One reason is to punish themselves if they feel bad about things or themselves. Most commonly, young people describe a feeling of relief or release with cutting, which means they don't have to concentrate on whatever was worrying them. Of course, it hurts, that is the point, because the physical pain gives them a focus which is outside of the other worries that are threatening to overwhelm them. The physical pain forces them to focus on that very immediate pain, and this may be the only way they have found to escape from the emotional pain that they are feeling the rest of the time. For those who overdose on tablets, the feeling of release is not there, but they are still getting away from the emotional pain by losing consciousness. All of them will see this as taking control over a situation over which they otherwise feel they have no control.

There are plenty of young people who will try self-harm, because they know of friends who do it, or they have seen it on the internet, and find it doesn't work for them, but some (maybe ten per cent of young people) will adopt this as a coping strategy in the absence of anything else that works for them. For healthcare professionals and parents, and for family and friends, the task then is helping them to find better coping mechanisms to deal with whatever worries, anxieties or fears they have.

'Pain works. Pain heals. If I had never cut myself, I probably wouldn't still be around today. My parents didn't help me, religion didn't help me, school didn't help me but self-harm did. And I'm doing pretty well for myself these days. Don't get me wrong, not in a heartbeat do I think that self-harm is a good or positive thing, or anything besides a heart-breaking desperate act that saddens me every time I hear about it. But there is a reason why people do it.

Young person, quoted in 'Truth Hurts'

As we have noted, this can only be done by addressing the under-lying problems, and young people may be very reluctant to discuss what those worries and anxieties are. Establishing a trusting relationship is key for healthcare professionals, for parents the hardest and most important thing may be to accept that actually you may not be the best person for your child to talk to initially. Opening up and admitting that you have a problem that you can't overcome alone is tremendously difficult for adults, and even more difficult for most young people. If there are complicating factors such as child abuse, where they know there will be tremendous impact on the family relationships, this is even harder. For most young people finding the right person to open up to is hard, especially when many adults are wary of opening the proverbial 'can of worms'. If you are a teacher, a healthcare professional or social care professional then it is important that, however busy our lives are, we see it is a privilege and an honour that a young person chooses to open up and share their worries with us. It means they have seen something in you that deserves their trust.

Alternatives to self-harm and suicidality?

What can be done to give young people back the feeling of control, and better ways of coping? The answers to this are best split into short- and longer-term solutions (with maybe one intermediate one!) It is very important that the short-term safety measures are not the only things put in place, but that they are used alongside a longer term approach to tackling the underlying issues that are leading to the symptom of self-harming. Elsewhere in this book we will have mentioned the problem of simply squashing one way of coping without putting in a better way of dealing with painful emotions. This usually just leads to another, different, set of symptoms, rather than everything just going away...

Short-term solutions

Some emphasis will be put by health professionals, particularly if there is some suicidal intent, on safety planning. In extreme cases, where safety cannot be guaranteed, hospital staff will want to keep children and young people at the hospital to ensure they do not continue to hurt themselves, and this may involve safeguarding procedures, or admission to a young person's specialist mental health in-patient unit. Either of these should be seen as a positive step, rather than a negative one; they won't be considered unless they are really needed, and if they are offered then it will be because the professional helpers think this is the best way to get longer term help for the individual.

More often safety planning might involve a temporary removal of sharp objects or access to medications within the home or residential setting to help overcome the impulse to self-harm. This can be problematic, because we have seen that control is important to young people, and effectively this further removes control. So plans like this need to involve the young person and be seen by them as a short-term aid while they move on to longer-term solutions. Simply removing the means to self-harm, without also starting longer-term solutions, will only lead to the young person looking for alternative means to self-harm.

The other aspect of short-term help is to install some other ways of reacting to the feelings that lead to self-harm. These usually take the form of distraction techniques: a lot of self-harm urges are impulsive, so finding alternative things to do while the urge is strong allows time to pass and the urge to go. In my experience this will work with relatively mild urges, and the key is to enable young people to find the thing that works for them. There are lots of resources online that give potential distractions, and some of them seem very facile or even ridiculous, but finding what works for the individual may take some experimentation with different things. Be careful what you search for online; there are some very negative sites which actually encourage self-harm, and these are obviously to be avoided. A couple of helpful and positive ones are included in the list at the end of this chapter.

Slightly different from distraction is the idea of substituting a mild stimulant to take the place of the painful effect of self-harm. Ideas such as using a rubber band around the wrist and snapping it against the skin to provide a very mild pain, fit into this category, and other ideas such as sucking ice cubes, or eating raw chillies also provide an alternative to cutting. These may not provide the answer, even a short-term answer, but they have some currency, and may work for some individuals in distress. From here it is a short step to the idea of 'harm reduction' which encourages a safe use of limited self-cutting, with hygienic sterile sharps. The theory is that this is safer than cutting with other implements which may lead to secondary infections and so on, and is a non-judgemental interim measure. It should only ever be considered as part of a much broader care package which is being run by an experienced mental healthcare professional. Even in that context it remains controversial, and many mental health staff will advise against it because of the risk of accidental injuries which may be far greater than intended.

Longer-term solutions

Longer-term solutions will depend on what is the underlying issue for the child or young person who is self-harming. For those who have anxieties or worries then addressing the worries will be the main concern, and it may be that the worries are related to something that we, as adults or parents, may consider as easily sorted out. Younger children who have a single teacher for a whole school year, for example, often get very anxious if they don't get along with that teacher and can't let them know what is worrying them. School based issues may be addressed by the parent talking to the school and clearing up misunder-standings, or getting arrangements changed. For many other worries and anxieties the rest of this book gives a range of different ways of addressing those worries, but the key will be in enabling the child or young person to initially be able to identify the source of the concerns, which they may not be able to verbalize, or may have difficulties in identifying themselves. The need to attend an emergency department and get a full assessment from a mental health professional may be the catalyst for beginning this longer-term approach to addressing the problems.

Intermediate solution: Cognitive Behavioural Therapy

Increasingly a form of Cognitive Behavioural Therapy (CBT) which focuses on coping strategies has been used with very good effect with young people who self-harm regularly. Dialectical Behavioural Therapy (DBT) can be used, usually in a group setting for young people, to look at dealing with the urges to self-harm and alternative strategies to cope with the emotions that drive these often-uncontrollable urges. Like CBT it focuses on the link between emotions and cognitions (thoughts) and the behaviours that follow, but is very much focused on giving new coping strategies for this particular issue. DBT is also used for other conditions in adults, but in young people it fits very well with overcoming self-harm urges, and where it has been used regularly it has reduced the rate of readmissions to emergency departments considerably. I've referred to it as an intermediate treatment because it is possible that the underlying issues will be resolved during the course of a series of DBT sessions, but if they are not, then DBT is not the only answer and other therapies will be needed to address those issues.

Parents' and other people's reactions – the emotional impact

This might have been a tough chapter to read. It is important to recognize our own emotional responses to self-harm in children and young people.

How can they do this to themselves?

Most of us would not consider harming ourselves, so it can be very difficult to put ourselves in the place of someone who has done. The physicality of the act can provoke a range of emotions, horror, revulsion, shock, even disgust, and may arouse feelings within helpers that they haven't fully processed themselves. Stigma around self-harm is deeply buried; there is some evidence that for some us there is a difference in how we perceive people who 'deserve' our compassion, and those who don't. The value-judgements that we make around this are deeply buried in how we are brought up to see the world, and although professional staff are trained to be non-judgemental, we are all human too, and without fully working through our own emotional responses it can be hard to put this into practice as much as we would like. For professional helpers in healthcare, social care and teaching, some reflection on how we work with this issue, and with similar issues which evoke emotional reactions, is important. Seeing the acts of self-harm as being a symptom of a deeper need, as a symptom of distress, is one way of revisiting these emotional responses. If they are able to inflict these wounds on themselves, or take that many tablets, how distressed must they be?

For parents, friends and family members the emotional response may be different because of the emotional attachment you have to that individual. Feelings of guilt that the young person has been distressed but not able to communicate their distress are common, but feelings of anger are equally common, as if the child's actions are somehow a reflection on their own failure 'to see this coming'. Alongside these feelings of helplessness and fear, there is a fear about how to cope if this happens again, of not knowing how best to react to these incidents. Resist the temptation to ask 'Why?' when you first find out about the self-harm; at this stage they may not be able to tell you why, and it adds to the pressure. Being there, and available to talk in a non-judgemental way, letting the young person know that you care, and you want to understand their individual feelings, and want to help, are the key things. While they may not be able to explain clearly how the emotions or anxieties are affecting them, it is also best not to try and guess what these are, or make assumptions about what is affecting them. Another part of growing up, despite the pressure to conform, is about establishing your identity as a unique individual, so assumptions that you know how they feel will often get a negative response.

This developmental context also explains the 'Why didn't they talk to me?' question. Growing older involves separation from dependency on your family and working towards independence. Talking to your parents may seem 'childish', and some young people seek to distance themselves from their parents' values and beliefs during this phase of their life, so a parent may the last person they want to talk to or open up to about their real feelings. This is painful for parents to experience, but the job of parents at this time of life is usually seen as just being there for them, and letting you love and care for them anyway. Professional staff who are trained to work with young people may be a more acceptable trusted person to talk to and provide help in the meantime.

A crisis such as an overnight (or longer) hospital admission and assessment can be very emotive, but it is also a good time to effect some change. The issues are suddenly out in the open and have to be talked about. Healthcare professionals have a distinct role, and as part of the assessment are allowed to ask difficult questions and address difficult issues. The safety and care planning may be the way that longer-term help is put in place, so although it is emotionally a difficult time, these crises are also opportunities to move forward.

Summary

Self-harm is an emotive and difficult subject, but it can provide the opportunity to put help in place. We have seen that self-harm is best understood as a symptom, often a symptom of distress or anxiety, so it needs to be taken seriously. A mental health assessment will help to determine how dangerous the self-harm is and point to the best long-term help, by therapies for anxiety or by addressing the other issues underlying the self-harm. Short-term measures can help the main symptoms, but getting help for the underlying issues is the key to moving forward.

References and further reading

Baldwin, L. (ed) (2020) Nursing Skills for Children and Young People's Mental Health. Switzerland: Springer, Switzerland.

McDougall, T., Armstrong, M. and Trainor, G. (2010) *Helping Children and Young People who Self-harm: An Introduction to Self-harming and Suicidal Behaviours for Health Professionals*. London: Routledge.

Mental Health Foundation (2006) *Truth Hurts Report*. Available at: <www.mentalhealth.org.uk/publications/truth-hurts-report1> (accessed 2 February 2021).

Online resources

Childline: <www.childline.org.uk> Childline will talk about all sorts of anxieties as well as self-harm urges. They have a special page on self-harm coping techniques: <www.childline.org.uk/info-advice/your-feelings/self-harm/self-harm-coping-techniques/>

Family Lives (formerly Parentline Plus):

Keep Your Head, Cambridgeshire & Peterborough C&YP Mental Health: <www.keep-your-head.com/cyp>

Harmless:

The Mighty, 21 Coping Skills for Self-Harm: <themighty.com/2019/06/coping-skills-self-harm/>

NICE   guidelines,   Self   harm: <www.nice.org.uk/guidance/condi-tions-and-diseases/mental-health-and-behavioural-conditions/self-harm>

Papyrus (Prevention of Young Suicide): <www.papyrus-uk.org>

Samaritans: <www.samaritans.org/> Primarily set up with adults in mind, but they do also work with young people.

The Mix, Self-harm coping tips and distractions: <https://www.themix.org.uk/mental-health/self-harm/self-harm-coping-tips-and-distrac-tions-5696.html>

Spun Out, Self harm distraction techniques: <spunout.ie/mental-health/self-harm/self-harm-distraction>

Young   Minds: <youngminds.org.uk/find-help/feelings-and-symptoms/self-harm/>

15

Managing anxiety in the family

Leah Benson, RMN & Systemic Practitioner

Managing anxiety as a family can be at times a real challenge, often having a significant impact on the family unit as a whole. In the following chapter we are going to look at how anxiety can affect the family, which may feel familiar to you, and how small changes can be made in the hopes of creating a real difference in your day-to-day lives. Families in the twenty-first century are often extremely busy with multiple competing factors. If your effort and hard work is focused on the right areas, it will hopefully improve both mental and emotional wellbeing for the family as a whole.

In order to tackle the difficulty it's important to have an understanding of the issue. If you haven't already done so, go back and look through Chapter 1. Having a good understanding of anxiety and how it could manifest in your child will help you to move forwards and implement changes to improve life. The key approach for the family is facing the fear and tolerating the distress in order to overcome the anxiety.

Anxiety is often described as infectious or as having a ripple effect within the family, creating difficulties for parents and children alike to manage and contain. As adults, having to support partners or children who are experiencing anxiety can often present a significant challenge. As parents, the burden to alleviate the distress of our children is immense and can lead to feelings of inadequacy and helplessness.

You may be wondering why we are thinking about the family in the context of anxiety. In therapy, family-based approaches can be offered as an intervention to support with anxiety problems or difficulties. These problems often show improvement when the family embraces a consistent and contained approach. The main focus is on relationships between people in families or wider extended networks who are felt to have significant roles. It aims to recognize the complex and multi-layered social systems that move a family from a position of stability to conflict or discord. If we can identify what these systems are, and understand their impact, a more harmonious and happy family can evolve.

One of the key areas that can go wrong or break down when families are in high states of worry or anxiety is communication. This might seem strange: don't we all communicate every day to some extent or another? But the key is to have effective communication. So how do we do this? It might be helpful to think about ways we communicate – verbal, nonverbal, written, or in other ways? And what our strengths are as individuals.

It's also important to remember that the art of effective communication is also in the listening. Children tend to respond, too, and will communicate their worries and anxiety in a multitude of different ways. We may notice small changes in their behaviour that can be easily dismissed as poor, naughty or confrontational. Here are a few ways in which children can express anxiety:

- High levels of distress and anger in small children.
- Regressing or exhibiting behaviours they have outgrown.
- Unhealthy eating or sleeping habits.
- Irritability in older teenagers and behaviours that could be described as acting out.
- Obstinate or uncooperative behaviours.
- Struggling with focusing on tasks or maintaining attention.
- Refusal to engage in hobbies or interests they used to enjoy.
- Physical pains that cannot be explained.
- Use of coping strategies such as substances or self-harm.

You may have recognized a few of these in your own child, but some you may not. This list is not extensive and all children are individuals and will express themselves as such. It is also important to remember that anxiety is not the driver for all behaviours, and at times children will become frustrated, uncooperative and irritable for reasons that aren't related to anxiety, just like the rest of us; these behaviours should be managed in the parenting approach you have agreed within your family unit.

Strategies and tips to think about

Speak plainly

When children are in a state of high arousal or distress it can be difficult for them to take in and understand what is being said to and asked of them. Try to speak as clearly as possible, communicate clear expectations and offer reassurance without allowing avoidance of the anxiety trigger. Try not to feed into the anxiety, and avoid repetition while ensuring the child has understood. This could be implemented when a child is repeatedly asking the same question in a particular situation (for example, if the child has a fear of dogs and being bitten). After you have answered their question clearly, if repetition occurs more than three times say you have already answered this question and ask your child to repeat back to you what your answer was.

Maintain calm

It is important to remain calm when responding to your child's worries or anxiety. This can be difficult at times, especially when your child is displaying high levels of distress. Remember you need to model to your child how to calmly respond to difficult situations. The hope is that your child learns how to cope and manage based on what they have observed you do ('learnt behaviour').

Keep a record of success

It is helpful for children of any age to see the progress they have made. Try keeping a diary or chart of your child's progress, their success, and when they have done well. Try and make this an interactive and engaging process and one that they can add to independently. Use it as a reference point for when things are more difficult. It is important to ensure that the diary is used consistently so it's relevant, and holds meaning for your child.

Positive language

Try to avoid negative language or conversation when progress is slow or blips happen that seem like setbacks. Try and remain positive, set goals and refer to the success chart or diary if you have one.

Routines

Try and ensure that you have, and maintain, a routine and structure to daily life but also one that helps you manage as a family in difficult situations. Try and ensure that these routines are adhered to, and try not to implement allowance or avoidance techniques – either from you or your children.

Picking battles

As parents, try to spend some time thinking about what the important boundaries are, and where allowances can perhaps be made. What is important to you as a family, and in raising your children? If as a family you are already under pressure managing day-to-day anxiety difficulties, it may be that allowances are made in other areas, or that in order to maintain parental resilience some rules become more fluid. This will help you to avoid constant and persistent conflict.

Pre-planning

Try to think ahead and be prepared for any possible triggers for anxiety-provoking experiences that you might encounter as a family on a day-to-day basis. This will help you to avoid being surprised or taken off-guard. It will also allow you to prepare your child and support them to think about strategies that may help them to manage their response to these triggers.

A place to put the worry

As part of your daily routine, set aside a time for listening to and discussing worries with your child. Try and keep this to a set time and do not overrun. Encourage your child to take their time and, as much as possible, avoid talking about worries outside of this allotted space. This time could be used creatively to write down the worries and place them in a worry box or other identified space that you place to worry into. This idea is once you have discussed the worry and addressed it you can then forget about it by writing it down and putting it away.

Consistency

As a family, discuss your expectations and how these can be adhered to. Make sure that all the house rules are clear, and maintain a consistent approach. It is important to take into account commonalities and differences, as this is key for siblings where age and developmental stages should be taken into account. A clear and consistent approach is helpful when trying to manage anxiety and can avoid conflict or avoidance. This can be similar to the managing reassurance section in Chapter 1 or building mastery and competence in Chapter 8.

Ellie

Ellie and her parents were seeking help for anxiety difficulties. In the first session they explained that Ellie had had difficulties with her anxiety for the past two years. Upon transitioning to secondary school things got much harder to manage. Ellie's mum explained during the session that she understands what Ellie is going through as she suffers from anxiety herself. She was keen to share her experiences with Ellie in the hopes that this would be helpful. Ellie's mum was described by the family as giving Ellie strategies and tips to help manage the anxiety. This, however, tended to cause arguments between the two of them. Ellie's dad, on the other hand, described feeling out of his depth and remained on the periphery of managing difficult situations.

Ellie's parents were taking vastly differing approaches to the situation. While it was clear that both parents wanted to help and support Ellie, with such a disparity of approach it was important to reach a shared understanding. We went back to basics to explore how they communicated as a family, talking and listening. It's important to remember that communication is not just verbal!

We talked through how the family were feeling during periods of increased difficulty or conflict. Ellie described feeling unsupported by her dad, and not listened to by her mum. This often escalated to arguments, high expressed emotions or feelings of isolation in the family home. 'High expressed emotion' is shorthand for a range of different emotions and behaviours, for example, anger and hostility, intolerance or criticism. This can often, understandably, be very unhelpful; however, it is a common place for families to find themselves in when managing prolonged periods of difficulty.

Ellie felt she was shouting at her parents a lot, and they agreed. It also transpired that all family members felt what they were doing was not 'good enough'. We talked through this common experience and feeling. The family were able to offer each other reassurance and gained a new perspective on how the others were feeling. This helped us to explore further how they as individuals experienced each other's behaviour, and what they could perhaps do differently.

Ellie's mum described feeling very surprised that Ellie did not feel listened to. We opened this up for the family to think about and it transpired that Ellie did not want her mum to share her own experiences, but to 'listen'. This felt like a real breakthrough for Ellie and her mum; they were able to think about how they could share and listen to each other's difficulties differently.

We explored Ellie's dad's role in the family, and he described at times feeling 'inadequate' when it came to helping. This would often lead to him avoiding situations or offering support. Both Ellie and her mum described this as being very frustrating. Ellie said she felt distant from her dad, and that he did not care. Her dad addressed Ellie directly and offered her assurance that he cared deeply for her and wanted to support her, but that he felt unsure about what to do for the best. He said he wanted to avoid conflict, and felt unable to help Ellie, or to make any difference to the situation.

This helped us to directly discuss what would be helpful at times of increased anxiety for Ellie. Ellie asked her dad to come and 'give her a hug' when she felt worried or distressed with her anxiety. We all agreed that this was something that he could certainly provide.

In the following sessions, Ellie's parents attended without her. We were able to explore and think about Ellie as a whole person outside of her anxiety difficulties. We discussed Ellie as a teenager experiencing significant hormonal changes as her body develops. It was important for the parents to gain a greater clarity of when/how to put in boundaries around behaviour. We explored defining and setting clear limits and boundaries, understanding how Ellie's anxiety may manifest itself but not accepting or tolerating the behaviour associated. Furthermore we talked about parental distress tolerance and the importance for parents to push Ellie with strategies.

After a number of sessions the family were reporting a significant reduction in conflict within the family unit. This provided them with a calm foundation to improve communication and support Ellie with managing her anxiety. The following key changes were made which provided maximum impact:

- Dad taking a more active role when difficult situations arose.
- Parents agreeing on a consistent approach and boundaries.
- Opening up lines of communication and 'how we listen'.

While all families are different, clear, calm and consistent communication is fundamental to addressing difficulties.

Advice for parents

Caring for a child who has additional needs such as anxiety can be stressful. It is a change to the normal parental role and requires an additional set of skills. It is normal for parents to feel a wide range of emotions when presented with a required shift in approach. Parents can often feel both emotional and physical stress as a result. Be kind to yourselves if you are feeling angry or frustrated with the situation: it is completely normal.

You may experience a number of the following emotions or feelings as a result of the increased stress and responsibility, and these could affect you in a number of ways; it may be helpful to look out for some of the following signs to monitor your own well-being:

- Worried and preoccupied by the situation.
- High levels of fatigue and irregular sleep pattern.
- Less tolerant (high expressed emotion).
- Low mood and sadness.
- Changes to appetite and physical body changes.
- Unexplained aches and pains or headaches.
- Loss of interest in hobbies or social events.

It is important as parents to recognize the demands of supporting a child with anxiety difficulties. As parents you may from time to time experience anxiety yourselves, or may struggle on a daily basis. It is important to ensure that support networks are built in to help with this and that you feel emotionally robust enough to manage this along with the other pressures of daily life. Do build a strong support network around you. This does not have to be in the traditional sense of extended family members or close friends; there are also lots of helpful online forums in order to access support. Families come in all shapes, sizes and structures. Whatever the make-up of your family, it is important to ensure that you have a consistent approach to parenting in general but also to specific issues that come your way. This can be draining and requires a great deal of resilience, both physically and emotionally. It is important to ensure that you prioritize your own needs which can sometimes be difficult to do. Below are some ideas that might be helpful to explore in building up parental resilience.

Ask for help

Identify family and friends who will be able to offer help and support. Structure what would be helpful from them and don't be afraid to ask. This may be as little as a non-judgemental ear to rely on when things are especially difficult.

Focus on your own health

It is important to try and maintain a balance for your own health and well-being. Ensure that you have taken the time to think about your own health needs and set goals for yourself. This may be time for exercise, sleep or similar activities. Of course, this may not always be possible, but even a small thing such as an online yoga session once a week can be helpful (see Chapter 2).

Connect with others

Seek out support groups either online or within your local community. They can help to provide validation and under-standing from those in a similar situation. These support groups can also provide valuable tips and strategies that are tried and tested to support you and your family.

Not just parents

As parents it can often be easy to lose your identity after having children and starting a family. It's important to ask the following questions to help support and equally balance the needs of all the family:

- What do I need?
- What do WE need?
- What does our FAMILY need?

These questions help to structure and prioritize shifting and competing demands without losing the importance of each.

References and further reading

Burnham, John B. (1986) *Family Therapy*, London: Tavistock.

Carr, A. (1997) *Family Therapy and Systemic Practice*, University Press of America.

Cecchin, G. (1987) *Hypothesizing, Circularity, and Neutrality Revisited: An Invitation to Curiosity*. Family Process, 26:405–413.

Dallos, R., & Draper, R. (2010). *An introduction to family therapy: systemic theory and practice* (3rd ed.).Maidenhead: McGraw Hill.

Pearce, W.B., & Cronen, V.E. *Communication, action and meaning: The creation of social realities*. New York: Praeger, 1980.

Vetere, A., & Dowling, E. (2005) *Narrative Therapies with Children and Their Families*. Routledge, London

Wilson, Jim (1998) *Child-Focused Practice*, London: Karnac.

16

Perspectives

Leanne Walker & Anais Bullock, experts by experience

Leanne Walker's story: managing anxiety

In this section, I will be writing about perspectives of managing anxiety, some of which come from my own lived experiences including reflections of being on waiting lists for support and what would have helped, knowing what I know now. Some come from what I have learnt from other children and young people, including friends, about what helps them. And some come from looking back and reflecting on what would have been helpful in managing my own anxiety. That's the thing – once lots of time and space has passed and you are not in that really difficult place anymore, you are able to look back on things differently and you reflect, often seeing things with a different perspective or clarity. And upon reflection, some of the things which would have helped are 'small' things, but do not underestimate the power of these, for sometimes it is these that can make the biggest difference.

Lived experience

I was about 14 when I first started to experience mental health difficulties including anxiety, that impacted my day-to-day life. I would be sitting in class at school and knots would begin to twist themselves inside my stomach, my palms would begin to sweat and yet my body wanted to shake as if it was cold, resulting in this slight tremble which felt like it was coming from my very core which I had no control over. Waves of dread and ripples of doom would swirl inside presenting as these intense physical symptoms. 'Is there something wrong with me?' I questioned myself. 'There's something seriously physically wrong,' I thought. I couldn't concentrate on the words the teacher was saying no matter how hard I tried; it was as if they were simply going straight over my head and I wasn't capable of taking them in. I wanted to be anywhere but where I was. Sometimes (if these feelings weren't rooting me to the spot), I would make my exit quietly as everyone was engaged in something else. I didn't want a fuss, I just wanted to – without anyone noticing – disappear into the emptiness of the bathroom as the knots twisted themselves into pain, and nausea added itself into the mix. Locked in the bathroom stall away from everything and everyone, I would find some kind of temporal relief as the intensity subsided somewhat.

Looking back now, I can so clearly see what I was experiencing as anxiety, but that's the thing – at the time I had absolutely no idea. I knew absolutely nothing about the symptoms of anxiety, including how it can affect the body; in fact I didn't know the first thing about anxiety and I'm not even sure I even knew the word anxiety existed, or if I did, it wasn't one I used within my own vocabulary. I was yet to connect the way in which mental health and physical health are related, and gave very little thought to my mental well-being in general. What I've learned from my own and from friends' experiences is that anxiety can present itself as any combination of a range of symptoms and can be triggered under an array of different circumstances. How anxiety presents for one person could be very different to another, and it doesn't need to mirror the experience of someone else exactly to be anxiety. I do not know your story, and of course this is only a tiny glimpse into mine, and there were many other factors shaping and influencing things for me as a young person experiencing anxiety. What I am trying to say is that what works for some, doesn't work for others, as personal situations differ and ultimately it's about finding what helps within your own personal circumstance. I want to note that I am not a mental health professional, I am just someone with lived experience of mental health difficulties, who has also experienced accessing, and trying to access, a range of mental health services.

Knowing about anxiety

For me, the important first thing about helping a child with anxiety is knowing about anxiety. As a parent or carer, take time to learn about possible signs and symptoms in children and young people, make sure to use reliable sites such as NHS (2019) and YoungMinds (2020). And secondly, talk to your child about it, and help them to understand, including the way mental health and physical health relate.

As a child or young person, not knowing what it is that you are experiencing can add to anxiety; it certainly did for me. A cycle of anxiety causing more anxiety. On that note, I think knowing that experiencing anxiety at times is a normal part of existence would have helped me, too. Anxiety is common, and lots of people struggle with it. At school, as I looked around at everyone else so seemingly carefree, I began to think it was just me.

In therapy, when I eventually did begin to talk about it and find the words to explain and understand what I was experiencing, I found it useful to use physical diagrams of people to consider how anxiety effects different parts of the body. I also found power in understanding why we even have anxiety in the first place, the role it plays within my own body, where it came from and how we have evolved. *It's not just me.*

Talking about it

It wasn't until I was at Child and Adolescent Mental Health Services (CAMHS) that I began to speak out loud about the symptoms I was experiencing. Up until then the intensity of it all lived inside my head (and showed outwardly as those physical symptoms I described at the start). Even now, stigma and fear can stop us talking about our mental health difficulties, but it's so important that we do. Speak to your child, show them it's okay to talk about it. Personally, for me, I didn't want my parents to do the whole 'sit down and seriously question me'; I preferred casual conversation, but you know your child best and what they are likely to respond to. *You are the expert in your own child.* Give your child room and space to talk and not be alone with what they are experiencing, without pushing them to talk if they don't want to. And if they don't want to talk, do remember that that is a choice, too. If they don't, make sure they know you are there if they do want to talk and also remember, things change, and, 'I don't want to talk about it' one week, doesn't necessarily mean, 'I don't want to talk about it forever.' Sometimes it may be that your child wants to let you know what's going on for them but physical words are too hard: perhaps try writing or texting to communicate instead as this also allows space to think about what you want to say to them. Or maybe they don't have the words to explain what they are experiencing, and drawing what they are experiencing could help them explain instead. Remember that for your child to engage in mental health services they have to be ready and willing. As a parent, you can feel ready and willing for them to engage but it may be they don't, and that can be frustrating but you can't force them to engage in support if they aren't ready, and having your support in whatever place they are in/what they choose to do, can make a huge difference.

Keeping a log

Once you and your child are aware of the symptoms of anxiety and how they may feel and present in their body, this makes identifying situations that increase anxiety (often called triggers) easier. At first, because I had no idea what anxiety was, I wasn't aware what was causing or triggering it. Looking back now, I am able to make connections, but at the time I didn't understand this at all and as I watched the minutes tick closer to the hour every day, I didn't know why this all-consuming doom swamped my body once again at the same time of day.

Something else some of my friends and I found helpful was keeping a written log about what was going on when experiencing anxiety. I started doing this at the start of Cognitive Behavioural Therapy (CBT) at CAMHS for my anxiety. Keeping a log of anxiety simply consisted of an A4 piece of paper marked into a grid with headings for 'time and date,' (when I started to experience symptoms), 'situation', (where I was and what I was doing), 'physical reactions' (where I would describe what was going on with my body), and 'thoughts' (where I would write anything I was thinking such as, 'I need to leave this situation'). This really helped me to discover themes: when I was experiencing anxiety; what was driving it, and this was important in helping me to begin working on managing it. You can find a similar sheet at Cornell University (2020). Or this is something you can do as a parent observing your child – an anxiety log sheet for this can be found at Understood For All Inc. (2020).

The words you choose are important

This may sound like a small thing but it had a big impact on me. Catching buses was one thing my anxiety eventually stopped me from doing. I would do everything to avoid them, often walking miles to places instead. Those around me didn't understand it and I don't blame them; at that time I didn't understand it either. I used to be able to get buses and then I couldn't any more, and I didn't have the words to explain why. 'It's just a bus, you used to get them'; 'stop being silly' – just some of what the people around me would say. My frustration turned inwards, I didn't want to be like this, I wasn't doing this for the fun of it. I wanted to be 'normal' and to just get on with my life like everyone else. As frustrating as it was for those around me, it was equally, if not more, frustrating for myself, and these comments only added to my negative feelings. Although something may seem small to you and you might not understand the anxiety or worry around it, try to understand it from your child's perspective – anxiety isn't something they can just switch on and off. I think it's very important to stay away from phrases that can invalidate feelings and shut down conversation. Even though sometimes these phrases come from a place of care as you don't want them to be experiencing what they are, just remember this is hard for them too. Your child might have an understanding why something is causing anxiety for them, but they might not, and therefore might not be able to explain their feelings to you and this could possibly come out as other feelings such as sadness and anger.

Support in the moment

Sometimes, that 'wave of dread' consumed me entirely and it felt like that was it for me, I would always be experiencing this and it would be my life forever and ever. Other times it felt like nothing outside of that moment of high anxiety existed as if the future was just a void of inexistence. What I have learned about heightened states of anxiety is that it passes; sometimes in the moment it felt like it wouldn't pass but it always has. Support your child in these moments. Reassure your child that they won't be feeling like this forever. Does a hug help them? Does just sitting with them help? Fiddling with something? I have found having some kind of fidget toy or something in my hands helps me. Remind them to breathe slowly and deeply. Often when I experienced intense anxiety, my breathing would quicken without me realizing and my hands would go all tingly and I'd feel like I was going to faint. Having people there for me and reassuring me that they weren't going to leave, not panicking and helping me until my anxiety reduced, helped me to manage these times.

On reflection, a simple breathing strategy could have helped me during this time such as counting my breaths, encouraging me to breathe slower, or modelling by doing this with me. As my breathing slowed down, the symptoms would often ease. Learning other techniques and strategies to help change the way your child thinks about their anxiety can also be helpful. Another technique I used was thinking of anxiety thoughts as a train. Visualizing standing at the station, I could hop on the train alongside the thoughts and see where it went (often with anxious or negative thoughts) or I could just watch the thought go by (if I did, it was then useful for me to do something else as a distraction).

Support groups

You can end up feeling very alone with all this stuff – I know I did for a while as a young person. I didn't understand myself so how could I expect other people to understand me? Having a space to share in this and learn and grow together can be helpful. Increasingly parent peer support groups are becoming established around the UK. These are spaces for parents to talk to other parents about their experiences such as what has been going on for them, what they find helpful to support their child, and some groups even put on different events. The Charlie Waller Memorial Trust (Charlie Waller, 2020) have developed a digital map which is updated regularly to show current parent peer support groups and organizations known to them around the UK.

There can be something powerful about speaking to others going through, or who have been through, similar experiences, learning and growing through these experiences together. It's important that you feel supported as a parent to be in the best position to help your child, to know you are not alone and not the only parent in the world experiencing what you are experiencing. Do some research and see what groups are in your local area that you could access. If my parents could have spoken to other parents going through the same thing I'm sure that would have been an invaluable source of support. For me as a young person, I was able to access a youth group with young people also experiencing mental health problems and it helped me so much knowing I wasn't alone with what I was experiencing, and that there were other people my age who understood me. I also made friends in this group, which has had a lifelong impact.

Ending thoughts

As a parent, wherever you are at, you are doing the best you can and sometimes you need to hear that. Remember that you know your child better than anyone else, and that includes professionals. At times it can feel like nothing will ever change and things won't get better, but they can, and they do. I think sometimes we can be too close to help and sometimes simply being there for your child and loving them unconditionally can be what they need from you.

Anais Bullock's story: warning signs of anxiety

Stress and anxiety are completely normal, however, when they stopped me doing the things I loved, it became apparent something was wrong. It's very hard to ask for help when you don't know what you need help with – this was always a struggle of mine. Trying to explain how overwhelmed I was beginning to feel was too challenging because no one else could see and I didn't know what was wrong. Anxiety is a protective factor (adrenaline and anxiety in humans is primarily for safety, for example, a caveman running away from a lion – fight-or-flight response), but nowadays our lives are very different; but our biology is the same.

So once panic attacks and avoidance became an everyday thing, my mum decided I needed some kind of support, whereas I was in denial, arguing it was a physical problem. When I think about the early days of being anxious, I never put the physical symptoms together as being anxiety, such as: stomach aches, frequent headaches, increased heart rate, dizziness, hair loss, fainting. I had countless doctor's appointments for the physical symptoms, but they were being caused by my anxiety and weren't the root of the problem. Symptoms that other people noticed included irritability, avoidance, leg bouncing, constant fidgeting, even specific things like fiddling with my earrings or pulling strands of hair out. At the time, most of these actions were subconscious, however if someone pointed them out to me, I would notice and then feel self-conscious, as this felt normal, and it felt uncomfortable for me to stay still. Now I can see that this was an automatic distraction technique to focus my brain on something other than the internal anxiety.

CAMHS have since helped me identify moments of anxiety during my childhood. One stood out a lot. I must've only been around seven and there was a talent show I was really looking forward to; however, when it came to the time to perform in front of a small audience, I got so worked up at even the thought of doing it, I was physically sick. This is one of my first memories of anxiety but was overlooked as a 'stomach bug' as I was so young and had never displayed this before. This is very relevant in my current anxiety as I fear being sick and will avoid social situations as a result. A main symptom of anxiety is nausea which really triggered that phobia for me, and as a result heightened my anxiety even more.

Triggers and environmental anxiety

Prior to my anxiety I had many interests such as gymnastics, which I attended two, three or four times a week, and competed in regional competitions, even winning some. For years gymnastics was my life and I really loved it, but as my anxiety increased I found myself avoiding sessions at the gym to the point of me going once a week, or driving there and having a breakdown in the car because I couldn't even force myself in. Going through the door was the most difficult part, however, when I was there within the first half an hour my anxiety had usually settled, but sometimes the anticipation and distress caused me to avoid going. Avoidance was the fuel for my anxiety; at the time it felt so hard to do something, and much easier to give in to not going, but this is what eventually helped my anxiety spill into every aspect of my life. It was really hard for me to give up gym, but all the enjoyment and passion was gone. Unfortunately, it became an additional pressure – it was no longer a happy place for me. On reflection it's such a shame, as I had many close friends and happy memories there and it's shaped parts of my personality. So, once my anxiety had taken gymnastics and that pressure was reduced, the focus for my thinking then became school.

Once again, like gymnastics, school was a happy place as I loved to learn and have always achieved highly despite my occasional self-doubt. The most difficult part of being anxious at school was that there was no break or relief from it. Silence in the lessons was the worst because my thoughts had no distraction and would completely overwhelm me. I was often unable to concentrate, which I had never struggled with before. Some of the thoughts would be completely irrational, like feeling everyone was staring at me or that I would choke and die if I didn't have a bottle of water with me at all times. These thoughts and many more would constantly be in my head and in turn pull down my mood. Days off school when I could not force myself in would be my only relief, but then the next day would come along and I was back to feeling the exact same – exhausted and anxious.

Anxiety lead into depression

For me, why the anxiety led into depression was due to feeling emotionally worn down. Being anxious a lot of the time naturally pulls your mood down, however when my anxiety became focused on my self-image, I began to feel very low. I started to see everything through a negative lens and my anxiety constantly focused on my every insecurity. It's like fighting someone who knows all of your weaknesses and how to use them against you. Evenings and times when I was by myself were particularly difficult. Due to anxiety I struggled with sleeping, which didn't help with my mood, but I was also up all night due to intrusive thoughts. Poor sleep paired with low motivation made getting out of bed a real struggle at times. When I look back now, I was starting to go down a dark path but was unaware. My favourite quote throughout my journey is that suicide is a permanent solution to a temporary problem.

What was helpful/not helpful at my lowest

My support system was key in me getting better and at the time staying safe. At CAMHS one of the most important things that helped was building a safe space to talk and a trusting relationship with my care co-ordinator, Kim. Kim really helped me communicate how I was feeling and when she understood it helped me validate my feelings, it made me feel so much less alone. My relationship with my mum and dad was strained as they were worried, and I didn't know how to reach out to them in case I worried them more. Kim bridged that gap and made me able to talk to my parents, and she explained what they didn't understand – this reduced my anxiety so much as she would start the conversation and the pressure wouldn't be all on me, especially with the difficult thoughts that I didn't want to always talk to my mum and dad about. One of the most important things Kim did was help my parents separate me from my anxiety, so as to detach it and not let it define me. It was us against my anxiety/depression. Kim also helped me explore different medications such as anti-depressants to try and lift my mood enough to try and work through my anxiety/depression. Kim also did CBT (Cognitive Behavioural Therapy) with me and helped me reframe my thoughts around school and myself, which I still use today.

Another person who really helped me was Emma, the outreach nurse who frequently saw me for an eight-week span at my lowest. The outreach team is an intensive community team that increases input at home or school when someone needs it. Emma came in at the perfect time as my mum was working full time and I was unsafe to be home alone, but having someone to talk to about my day when I got home was comforting and the support I received during that time was crucial. We went out a few times to Costa and that challenged my anxiety a lot, but having

Emma to talk those negative thoughts through whilst being in that situation was so helpful. Emma usually saw me at home as that was somewhere where I was comfortable, and sometimes at school, which got me through particularly tough days. When I felt that low, I didn't have any motivation, but seeing Emma and Kim every few days kept me encouraged to stay safe and gave me something to look forward to in the short-term future.

At school I had lots of support; Mrs Owen, Mrs Wood, Mrs Jones, but Mrs Cuthbert and Mrs Parnell in pastoral were my main support. They were both there when I was extremely anxious at school, Mrs Cuthbert and Mr Smith (with Kim) put lots of things in place within school to help such as an 'get out of lesson' card, arranged for me to drop geography to ensure I could catch up with my other subjects. They also decided, with my parents, to give me the responsibility to decide whether to attend each lesson and when I was at my most anxious, this took a lot of pressure off, as I found it tough to go to all six lessons back-to-back with no break from my anxiety. Mrs Wood was the teacher I would go to during my gaps from geography, she helped me with the work I needed to catch up with and kept me on track. Art was a really good distraction for me as, since I was a child, I have loved art, and Mrs Owen was always kind and definitely distracted me with her singing, dancing and positive attitude. Mrs Cuthbert and Mrs Parnell were so supportive when I was struggling, always had time to have a chat and made everything not seem so bad – even on my worst days they would make me smile. A big step for me was reaching out to someone at school.

My friends, Mum, Dad, sisters, Aunty Lynda and Uncle Martyn were a huge support system for me. My friends helped me through everything and even the little things like walking to school reduced my anxiety so much – most days they were the only reason I went to school. My relationship with my friends today is what got me through, they're all so amazing! My friends Beth, Holly, Lucy, Millie and Charlotte were there for me regardless of what was going on in their lives, which I'll never forget. My sisters were such a good distraction for me as they're little, and so happy, it made me forget how I was feeling. My Aunty Lynda, Uncle Martyn and mum would get me to go with the to the local pub quiz night, sometimes every week; this helped build my confidence and I used to have a really lovely time despite feeling anxious. Even if we have only come 3rd once, it's something I can't wait to be able to do after coronavirus has gone! My dad rings me every morning and every night since I don't get to see him every day; I love talking about our day, it helps a lot, especially in the morning as this is when I felt most anxious and he understands as he struggles with anxiety. I also used to ring my mum in school if I was anxious or upset, and she would always calm me down and help me get through it – this communication was vital as I reached out when I was struggling most, it reassured me I was okay. My mum and dad being unjudgmental and always accepting what I was feeling was the most helpful; sometimes a hug after a long day was all I needed.

During my lowest point my own unhealthy mechanisms were probably the most unhelpful – I know now I was just trying to control things I couldn't. Some medications such as fluoxetine and sertraline were unhelpful for me, but it's different for every person, what works for you might not for me, but Kim and I eventually found the right one. Personally I didn't find mindfulness very beneficial, but I think that's because I had a lack of motivation and couldn't see the point in it, or the point in getting better because I thought I was always going to feel like that, so I thought, 'why bother trying to change it?' Avoidance was helpful in the short term, but long term aided my anxiety and slowly I was trying to avoid everything even down to getting out of bed.

Recovery – how things started to get better

The most important thing I realized was that you can't get better unless you want to get better. In April 2020 my granny passed away and this made me think that she wouldn't want me to live like that and I decided that I wanted to get better for her – I wanted to be able to enjoy time with my family and friends again. This experience, even though painful, shifted my mindset toward recovery; it created a motivation to live life again, how my granny would've wanted me to. I learnt that people around me were my main help and that I had to reach out when I was struggling and that some of my 'coping mechanisms' were making things worse. Also, you have to celebrate the small victories like leaving the house twice in one day or spending more time with family. And don't be so critical of yourself – you're trying your hardest and the people you may compare yourself to could be going through the same things, but all you can see on the outside is a smile. Accepting that you have gone or are going through something helps you move on. And on a bad day I try to remember not every day is good, but there is good in every day.

Reflections

Going through this made me so much stronger as a person and helped me learn a lot about myself, and I can now recognize when I'm not doing too good and what I can do to feel better. At the beginning I was really fearful of feeling anxious, but now it doesn't control me and that's the difference – giving in and avoiding something just hands over more control, but to try and get better you have to try and push through it. As my mum would always say, no matter how hard it feels, it's never as bad as your mind is telling you. Since pushing through my anxiety, I have been to London on a train, been on a plane and have had my first job interview – I'm even enjoying sixth form. Six months ago, I wouldn't have even imagined doing any of that, I would've had a panic attack thinking about going on a flight! I'm really glad I got the opportunity to write this, as it's helped me look back and see how far I've come, but also, I hope that my struggles might be able to help someone else. Things can get better, you have lived through your worst day and there will be more, but there will be lots more amazing days – live for the good days you haven't had yet, not the bad.

References and further reading

Charlie Waller (2020) *Parent Support*. Available at: <charliewaller.org/parent-support> (accessed 17 October 2020).

Cornell University (2020). Anxiety Tracking Log. Available: at: <health.cornell.edu/sites/health/files/pdf-library/anxiety-tracking-log.pdf> (accessed 17 October 2020).

NHS (2019) *Anxiety in Children*. Available at: <www.nhs.uk/conditions/stress-anxiety-depression/anxiety-in-children/> (accessed 17 October 2020).

Understood For All Inc. (2020). *Download: Anxiety Log to Find Out Why Your Child Gets Anxious*. Available at: <www.understood.org/en/friends-feelings/managing-feelings/stress-anxiety/download-anxiety-log-to-find-out-why-your-child-gets-anxious-or-stressed> (accessed 17 October 2020.

YoungMinds (2020) *Anxiety*. Available at: <youngminds.org.uk/find-help/conditions/anxiety/?gclid=EAIaIQobChMItoGEicS77AIVF-DtCh3Y-VwaQEAAYASAAEgJ-D_D_BwE.> (accessed 17 October 2020).

Index